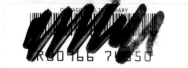

PLAYING IT SAFE

PLAYING IT SAFE

Milady's Guide to Decontamination, Sterilization, and Personal Protection

Sheldon R. Chesky

Isabel Cristina

Richard B. Rosenberg

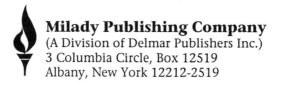

Milady Publishing Company
(A Division of Delmar Publishers Inc.)
3 Columbia Circle, Box 12519
Albany, New York 12212-2519

NOTICE TO THE READER

Publisher: Catherine Frangie
Developmental Editor: Joseph Miranda
Production Manager: John Mickelbank

Full Production: Gamut Production
Freelance Project Editor: Cynthia Lassonde

© 1994 Milady Publishing Company
(A Division of Delmar Publishers Inc.)

For information address:
Milady Publishing Company
(A Division of Delmar Publishers Inc.)
3 Columbia Circle, Box 12519
Albany, NY 12212-2519

Printed in the United States of America
Published simultaneously in Canada
by Nelson Canada,
a division of The Thomson Corporation

1 2 3 4 5 6 7 8 9 10 XXX 00 99 98 97 96 95 94

Library of Congress Cataloging-in-Publication Data

Chesky, Sheldon R.
        Playing it safe: Milady's guide to decontamination, sterilization, and personal protection/Sheldon R. Chesky, Isabel Cristina, Richard B. Rosenberg.
        p. cm.
        Includes bibliographical references and index.
        ISBN 1-56253-179-4
        1. Beauty shops—Sanitation. 2 Beauty shops—Employees—Health and hygiene. I. Cristina, Isabel. II. Rosenberg, Richard B. III. Milady Publishing company. IV. Title.
RA617.C48   1994
363.11'964672—DC20   93-36024
                                                                              CIP

CONTENTS

CHAPTER FOUR

Breaking the Chain of Cross-Infection 29

CHAPTER FIVE

Decontaminating Materials and Procedures 39

CHAPTER SIX

Sterilization 63

APPENDIX C

Characteristics of
Particles and Particle Dispersoids 99

INTRODUCTION

The History of Decontamination

When your clients enter the salon, they automatically assume the salon is clean and free from germs. Your customers also assume you and your co-workers have properly disinfected all equipment and environmental surfaces. Your clients assume they will not be exposed to infectious agents, which may possibly make them sick or, perhaps, even cause death as a result of your services.

We generally assume our clients are free from contagious agents (germs). We perform a variety of cosmetic services routinely touching the clients' skin. Occasionally, one might even accidentally nick or puncture a client's skin, resulting in slight bleeding, or one might cut or nick one's own skin causing bleeding. Either way, an open *port of entry* for germs is created.

Further, some treatments, such as electrolysis, whirlpool therapy, manicures, facials, or deep skin cleansing, might result in exposure to a client's mucous membranes, other body fluids, or exposed tissues. When you are cleaning the treatment equipment (scissors, razors, nippers, tools, tables, electrolysis devices, tubs, spas, or baths), you are exposing yourself to a variety of microbes. Thus, you are at risk of exposing yourself to a variety of infectious agents, first, when administering to your client, and, second, when cleaning up and preparing for your next client. Finally, if the cleaning and decontaminating process is not done properly, both you and your clients are at considerable risk of exposure to infectious agents, which are capable of getting both of you sick.

The purpose of this book is to help you protect yourself and your clients from infectious agents and the potential illnesses they may cause as a result of being exposed to or contaminated by these agents. This text is structured for the reader to learn about the principles of decontamination, sterilization, and personal protection in an easy-to-understand, easy-to-learn format.

This book is also intended for those readers who wish to have a practical guidebook on decontamination and cleaning of salons in the beauty industry.

The objectives of this book are:

- To make the reader fully aware of the sources of contamination, (namely, people, products, and the environment).

- To provide the reader with a basic background and understanding of the types of contamination that may be present in the salon.

- To help the reader understand the difference between cleaning and killing microbes.

- To familiarize the reader with the steps needed to achieve proper cleaning and decontamination in a salon.

- To educate the reader (whether a student, experienced beautician, technologist, or owner) on the most current methods of cleaning and decontaminating the equipment, tools, and environmental surfaces present in a salon.

- To acquaint the reader with the legal and governmental regulations relating to decontamination.

- To reinforce the need for proper personal hygiene.

- To provide the reader with a practical, hands-on guide for good salon practices for decontaminating all surfaces that could create an unsafe environment.

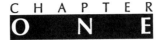

A Historical Look at Germs

❏ **LEARNING OBJECTIVES**

After completing this chapter, you should be able to:

■ Understand the history of the spread of common germs and the diseases they cause.

■ Define the fundamental rule for the protection of you and your clients.

■ Explain why it is important to be responsible for keeping the work environment clean and safe from germs.

■ Identify areas and situations in the salon that provide a risk of contamination and cross-infection.

Introduction

Since the beginning of recorded time, humanity has had to deal with germs. Even though people living thousands of years ago had no real concept of an invisible world of living organisms capable of getting them sick or possibly causing death, several references to diseases caused by these organisms (germs) are found in the Bible. As a matter of fact, the first infection-control rules for preventing the spread of disease are mentioned in Leviticus, a Biblical text. People afflicted with **Hanson's disease**, also known as **leprosy**, were removed from the general population and isolated into colonies away from the general public to keep the disease from spreading. Their clothing, possessions, and dwellings were burned to prevent the spread of the disease-causing organism, even though no one at that time knew the cause of the illness. Today we know leprosy is caused by a bacterium in the same family as the bacteria that causes **tuberculosis** (*mycobacteria tuberculosis*).

Throughout history, this phenomenon of epidemics, death, burning of possessions, and isolation was repeated. In the Middle Ages the Plague ravaged most of Europe. Approximately one third of the population died from *yursinia pestis*, the microorganism (bacteria) responsible for the disease. A statue in Vienna commemorates the human suffering for which the Plague was responsible. (Figure 1–1.)

Cholera and typhoid fever have been the scourges of many societies as have many other diseases. Currently, there is a

FIGURE 1–1
This statue in Vienna commemorates the Plague caused by the bacteria *yursinia pestis*.

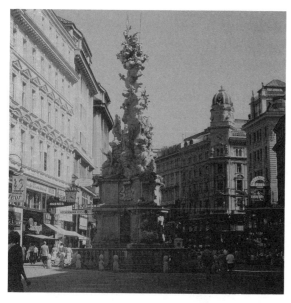

cholera epidemic throughout Central and South America. Typhoid fever, thought to be eradicated, is still present in many of the underdeveloped nations of the world.

Fortunately, we do not have to deal with the magnitude of the great Plague's devastation, although ancient diseases, such as cholera and typhoid fever, still emerge. We are faced with more modern-day problems concerning the spread of common germs and the diseases they cause. Even though many of the microorganisms we now deal with are different from past ones, the struggle goes on to identify, to investigate their spread, and to break the chain of cross-infection that still remain. For example, tuberculosis, which was predominant in the Dark Ages, still causes problems, including death. There are newer, more drug-resistant strains of this bacterium. Many of the more common germs present throughout history, such as *staphylococcus, streptococcus,* and many others are still responsible for infections causing death if improper treatment is given, or if a patient's immunity systems fail. And even more important, common-sense steps of prevention should be practiced to prevent the spread of diseases, providing personal protection against infection. This now becomes an important issue for both you and your clients.

The germs we may be exposed to have been around for a long time, having managed to survive an array of attacks. By following adequate cleaning practices with proper infection-control techniques, you will certainly protect yourself and your clients. The fundamental rule "clean and disinfect to protect all," is the basis for this text. If you do not know your clients are sick, you would not know whether or not your clients are carriers of germs, making you vulnerable to their germs. Even more, if you do not do a good job of decontaminating your work station and equipment, you could be the source of cross-infection from one client to another, spreading diseases without them or you knowing it.

It has taken people thousands of years to realize proper cleaning and disinfecting are absolutely necessary for human life to continue. To inadvertently spread germs from one person to another contributes to epidemics such as the flu, measles, mumps, herpes, and a myriad of other diseases including hepatitis, often referred to as the modern-day version of the Plague.

Who Is Responsible for Sanitization?

You are responsible for keeping the work environment clean and safe from soils and germs. You are not asked to keep your work area as clean as a hospital operating room, but it would be a good idea to try to keep your area almost as clean. Hospitals know how to keep germs from spreading. All of us share a mutual responsibility to assure our environment is clean and safe to live and work in; but once again, you are responsible to make sure your implements and all surfaces (e.g., tools, combs, brushes, countertops, chairs, mirrors, floors, sinks) are free from the possible contaminants that could get you and your clients sick.

Why? Simply because of good common sense. When clients see a messy work station, they might assume your work will be just as unkempt. They also might assume you are not doing a very good job of keeping your implements clean and free from microorganisms. As more of the general public becomes aware of how diseases are spread, they demand to know if the right steps to protect them from diseases are being followed by many different occupations, including yours.

Only you can determine if you have properly decontaminated your work area and implements. If brushes, combs, and scissors look dirty, you know they are dirty. If you can see soils, you can assume there is microbial contamination present also. The things you cannot see with the naked eye may hurt you and your clients. If you clean your work area and tools but neglect to disinfect your work area, all you have done is diluted the germ population, not removed it. Some cleaning agents might even be a growth medium for germs. It is well know most bar soaps will support the growth of microorganisms rather than kill them. This is why liquid hand soaps dispensed from a pump are pre-ferred, especially those containing an antimicrobial agent.

What do you do with scissors contaminated with a client's blood if you accidentally nick someone? How do you treat razors used for shaving or trimming once they have cut a client's skin? How do you protect yourself while protecting your clients from the possible blood-borne germs (called **pathogens**) present on these implements?

This book will provide you with the background necessary to handle these and many other situations dealing with personal protection and decontamination. The *principles of cleaning and decontamination* are the essential building-blocks providing you and your customers the protection from the risk of cross-infection. In order for you to have a working understanding of these principles, you must have a basic knowledge of organisms that cause disease in people and how these organisms are spread. (Figure 1–2.)

FIGURE 1–2
A microscopic view of various organisms.

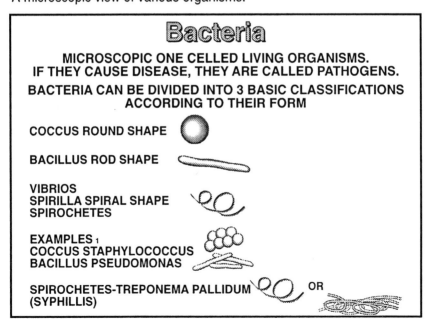

❏ REVIEW QUESTIONS

   1. Name the microorganisms (bacteria) responsible for the
   death of approximately one third of the population
   during the Plague of the Middle Ages.

   2. What is the fundamental rule for the protection of cosmetologists and clients against germs?

   3. Who is responsible for sanitization in the work place?

   4. Why is liquid soap dispensed from a pump preferable to
   bar soap for general use in a salon?

   5. What do the principles of cleaning and decontamination provide for cosmetologists and clients?

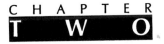

The Microbial World

❑ **LEARNING OBJECTIVES**

After completing this chapter, you should be able to:

■ Define microbiology.

■ Discuss the general types of microorganisms, where to find these microorganisms in the environment, as well as on or in people, and the conditions for growth and survival of these organisms.

■ Understand and become familiar with the terminology used in microbiology.

■ Discuss the impact microbes play in our daily lives.

Introduction

The advances of science and technology have provided the ability to identify and understand what causes most diseases and how to prevent their spread. The science of *microbiology* has been the primary resource to achieve this understanding. Microbiology provides the medical community with the knowledge necessary to treat diseases. Without microbiology, medical doctors would lack the modern skills to treat diseases, and public health departments would still insist on burning dwellings and possessions in order to prevent epidemics.

This chapter is designed to familiarize you with microbiology, so you may have a basic understanding of the microbial world and how it affects your job. Your understanding of the principles of microbiology and how germs grow and spread will help you make your world a safe environment.

What is Microbiology?

Microbiology is the branch of science studying the microbial world. Essentially, microbiology is devoted to the study of living organisms unseen by the naked eye. These organisms are called ***microbes*** or ***microorganisms***. As the names imply, in order to see and study microbes, microscopes or other kinds of magnifying devices are necessary. (Figure 2–1.) This science is relatively young with most discoveries occurring in the last 100 years, even though the first microbes were seen in 1675 by Antony van Leeuenhoek, the father of the microscope.

FIGURE 2–1
Microscopes are essential to the study of organisms.

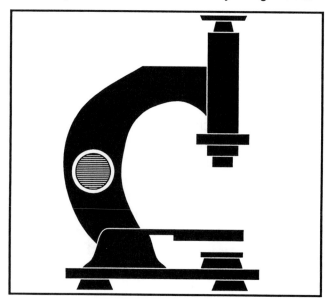

In the 1800s, several notable scientists began to use the newly-invented microscope to learn the cause-and-effect relationship among microbes, mostly concerned with human and animal diseases. Oliver Wendell Holmes, a famous Supreme Court Justice and physician, and Ignaz Semmelweis, a noted surgeon, are given credit for demonstrating the spread of diseases from skin-to-skin contact by hands and from clothing. Other great scientists of the times made discoveries demonstrating the disease-causing effects of certain microbes, and suggested ways to reduce or eliminate the spread of these contagions.

Dr. Louis Pasteur disproved the theory of spontaneous generation of disease. Invisible microorganisms, Pasteur demonstrated, had to be present in order to cause disease. Pasteur's work is credited for saving the French wine industry by discovering a process known today as ***pasteurization***. Pasteurization heats materials to a temperature destroying most of the microbes, but not all of them. Pasteurization is not appropriate for use in a salon for several reasons, mostly since you will want to destroy all growing organisms, not just most of them.

Dr. Joseph Lister and other scientists were instrumental in discovering chemicals to reduce the risk of infection caused by the transfer of germs from one person to another. These agent were developed to ***decontaminate*** or to kill the microbes responsible for causing an untold number of deaths. Lister distilled a chemical from coal tar called carbolic acid, also known as ***phenol***, to wash his surgical instruments, patients' skin, the operating table, and his own hands. Lister used bandages and dressings soaked in phenol. The results of using phenol demonstrate a surprising fact: When phenol was not used, most surgical patients died after surgery; but when phenol was used, many of the patients survived.

At the same time, another group of medical scientists in France and Germany began to use bleach (*hypochlorite*) as both an antiseptic and as a decontaminating agent. These scientists used the hypochlorite solution the same way Lister did, applying these chemicals to many surfaces, including wound surfaces directly.

The scientific community began to realize one person could infect another person with germs, and so, the germ theory evolved. The germ theory states *germs*, living particles that cause disease, are capable of spreading from one person to another. Germs present in body secretions, blood, and excrement from people who are sick can be transferred to other people who are not sick, thereby infecting them. Furthermore, there might be people who carry these particles, but do not show any symptoms or signs of illness. These *carriers* are capable of transferring germs. This theory was responsible for opening the door to the knowledge we currently possess on the origin, identification, and spread of diseases.

Microbiology has been the cornerstone of modern medicine. Without the advances in this science, many of the common, easy-to-treat illnesses would still be fatal to a great number of the population, leaving humanity without the basic knowledge to prevent the spread of germs. Microbiology is important to you because this knowledge will help protect you and your clients from germs.

The work of Dr. Joseph Lister, Dr. Robert Koch (the scientist developing many of the methods and techniques used to study microbiology today), and many others have given us the background to learn and protect ourselves from harmful microbes present in our daily living.

General Description of Microbes

The microbial world consists of many different life forms. First and foremost, microbes are extremely minute living particles requiring magnification to see them. Microbes come in various shapes, sizes, and can live in the most extreme environments on the planet. Microorganisms are found from the Arctic Circle to the vents that release the gases from underwater volcanoes. Microorganisms are found in the air we breathe, and there are microorganisms surviving without air. Plainly stated, microbes are found everywhere on earth.

Microorganisms may be classified as either plants (bacteria), animals (protozoans), or they assume forms of life such as viruses, fungi, or other types of microscopic life.

For your background information, this text deals with the more common forms present; the ones with which you should be concerned. (Figure 2–2.)

FIGURE 2–2
Microbial contaminants of our environment.

GRAM POSITIVE BACTERIA

GRAM NEGATIVE BACTERIA

ACID FAST BACTERIA

FUNGI, MOLDS, YEASTS, ENDOSPORES, LIPOPHILIC VIRUSES, CHLAMYDOSPORES

PROTOZOA, WORM OVA

Bacteria

Bacteria are one-cell plants. Most bacteria do not contain *chlorophyll*. Chlorophyll is the substance that makes plants green. It is the key compound in photosynthesis. A single bacterial cell is called a ***bacterium***. The plural form is called ***bacteria.***

There are bacteria living in oxygen-rich environments (such as air) called ***aerobic bacteria***, and there are bacteria needing no air called ***anaerobic bacteria***.

Bacteria are also classified by their shape. Their shape may become part of their name, giving clues as to their composition. A round or marble-shaped bacterium is referred to as a ***coccus*** (the plural is ***cocci***). An example of the use of coccus is *streptococcus*, as in *streptococcus faecialis,* the organism responsible for causing strep throat. Other organisms having the same characteristic shape are the *staphylococci*, such as *staphylococcus aureus*, which is responsible for staph infections. Staphylococci grow in clumps, and under the microscope they look like a cluster of marbles. When they infect the skin, you cannot tell what you are dealing with because they may resemble an open cut.

Some bacteria are rod-shaped. They are referred to as ***bacillus*** (the plural form is ***bacilli***). A great number of kinds of bacteria have this shape. *Pseudomonas*, a bacteria present in most tap water, has this shape. So does the organism causing tuberculosis (*mycobacterium tuberculosis*).

Another bacterial shape is the spiral, known as ***spirochetes***. Under the microscope these organisms look like little corkscrews. One of these organisms is responsible for causing syphilis (*treponema pallidum*).

Modern microbiology uses the gram stain technique to help see these microbes when examining them under the microscope. The staining technique is a primary method of further identifying these organisms since some will be colored blue (gram positive organisms) and some will be colored red (gram negative organisms). Although the staining technique is commonly used, you should know there are other microbial staining techniques used to help make the organisms visible under the microscope. Without these staining techniques, we still would have great difficulty seeing these organisms, even with the most powerful microscopes.

Reproduction and Growth

Bacteria reproduce through a method called **binary fission**. Simply stated, when bacteria reproduce, they split in two. This is why it is referred to as binary fission, or "the making of two by splitting in half."

A bacterial spore is a survival form for only some types of bacteria when conditions for growth become intolerable. It is not a means of reproduction. Bacterial spores may be produced when the temperature, moisture, or other necessity for active life of the bacteria becomes so adverse that the active form of the bacteria, called the **vegetative** form, can no longer survive. Remember, not all bacteria produce spores, nor are spores means of reproduction. Bacterial spores only allow the species to survive. Importantly, bacterial spores are not fungal spores.

Some bacteria produce materials to ensure their ability to survive the daily rigors of living. For example, the *pseudomonads* (responsible for several types of infections) make a slimy outer coating that keep the cell moist and protect the cell from drying out. The *tuberculosis bacillus*, a rod-shaped microbe, has a hard outer waxy coat to protect it from drying out as it floats in the air. Tuberculosis is generally spread by inhaling droplets of air. The bacteria are suspended in it. We will cover how diseases are spread in the next chapter.

Since bacteria surround our very existence, we are constantly exposed to microorganisms. Bacteria live on our skin, in our bodies, on our clothing, on work surfaces, and just about everywhere else, unless we take steps necessary to stop their growth. Under ideal growth conditions, the typical bacteria will reproduce every 12–15 minutes. For example, if we started with a one-cell organism and all its descendants survived at the end of a 24-hour period, we would be left with 100,000,000,000,000,000,000,000,000,

000,000,000,000 cells (1×10^{38}). Fortunately there are many reasons why this will not occur; but if we did not take the steps necessary to either prevent or remove the bacteria, they would continue to multiply. When you smell something rotting, you can be sure bacteria are hard at work.

Approximately 2,000 species of bacteria have been identified and about 10 billion would fit on the head of a dime. It would take roughly 30 trillion bacteria of average size to weigh an ounce.

Structure of Bacteria

As mentioned earlier, bacteria are single-cell plants. They have a distinct cell wall, a nucleus containing the genetic code, cytoplasmic constituents filling the cell (its "guts"), a possible way of moving around (a tail or a whip called a **flagellum**), and anchoring strands (**fimbri**) allowing the bacteria to hold on to an object. Figure 2–3 shows the loca-

FIGURE 2–3
The structure of bacteria.

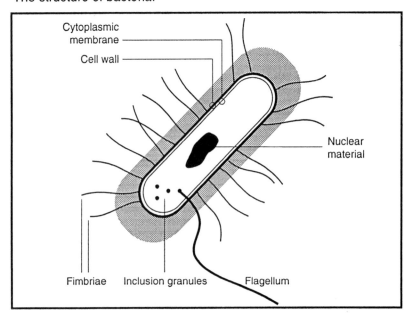

tion of these structures. Later, when we review the steps needed to decontaminate, we stress cleaning with a little "elbow grease," that is, applying pressure as you scrub. We recommend this so you will help break the hold of the fimbri, thus allowing removal of the bacteria.

Fungi

Fungi, (the singular is *fungus*), are a diverse group of living organisms found throughout the world. There are macrofungi and there are microfungi forms. An example of a macrofungus we have commercialized is the mushroom. An example of commercially used microfungi are the yeasts used for making bread, cheese, beer, wine, and alcohol. Without the use of these commercially important fungi, the world would be a very different place than it is today. There would be no breads, tofu, wine, beer, spirits, soy sauce, or antibiotics. That's right: antibiotics were first produced from fungal sources. The penicillins, cephalosporins, and others are derived from fungi.

Description

Microfungi share many similarities with the lower forms of plants and animals; however, fungi are not closely related to either, even though they are considered part of the plant kingdom. They have distinct rigid cell walls. Animal cells do not have cell walls; they have flexible cell membranes. This is one of the distinguishing characteristics between plants and animals. Fungi are *multi-cellular*, which means they are made up of many cells. The fungi can be separated into two general groups: yeasts and molds. Refer back to Figure 2-2. for an example of what microscopic fungi look like. Notice the strand-like appearance.

Fungal infections are a significantly troublesome group of infections, ranging from classic skin problems to deep-seated respiratory infections, sometimes killing people. The classic yeast infections (nail fungus, ringworm, athlete's foot, jock itch, and a variety of other diseases) all have fungal sources. Many of the skin rashes you will be exposed to in your career will be caused by fungi. Care should be exercised when you encounter skin rashes, since many of them may be contagious and easily transmitted. It is essential proper cleaning and decontamination steps are used if you are to provide a safe work environment free from most of these fungal sources.

Growth and Reproduction

Fungi live almost everywhere. They are as common as bacteria. They feed on everything from dead tissue to living cells, including skin. Most fungi prefer a somewhat moist environment, but this is not necessarily true all of the time. Many molds like the warm dry environment of the desert. When these infect the lungs, a disease called desert fever may result.

Fungi reproduce both sexually and asexually. Yeasts form buds, break off from the mother and grow into adults.

Fungi can enter the body without breaking the skin. Athlete's foot is spread by walking on a surface having been contaminated with fungal spores. These spores attach themselves to intact skin and begin to grow. The result is a highly irritated area with itching and burning. Fortunately, there are many good over-the-counter drugs effectively controlling this infection. Note fungal spores differ from bacterial spores. Fungal spores are used to spread the species and are a form of the reproductive cycle; whereas the bacterial spore forms only to survive.

Viruses

Of all the forms of life the **virus**, or viral particle, is the smallest complete form of life. It is a true parasite, having to invade a cell and use it for nutrients in order to survive and reproduce. Viruses were discovered about 100 years ago and are extremely small. By comparison, bacterial cells are 100-story buildings compared to a grain of sand representing a viral particle.

Viral particles are spread by a variety of ways. They may hitchhike on a dust particle or inside a bacterial cell. They may be on a droplet of saliva when someone sneezes or coughs. They may be deposited on an inanimate object like a countertop or scissors. They may be on the door handle to your shop or on the handle of your clippers. You will never know if viral particles are present, but when disease strikes you or one of your co-workers, you will know they were present.

Viruses are the source of the common cold, influenza, measles, chicken pox, mumps, herpes (cold sores and genital varieties), polio, infectious mononucleosis, Hepatitis B virus (HBV), and HIV-1 (the AIDS virus). An environmental surface has a direct correlation to the chain of transmission with many of these viruses. The common cold, influenza, and some other respiratory viruses are commonly spread by hand-to-surface-to-hand contacts. Other viruses require the particles be transferred from one person to another through more direct routes, including through the transfer of blood or body fluids. Dirty, contaminated instruments containing blood or body fluids have been linked to the spread of the AIDS virus.

Animal Microbes

The animal kingdom contributes its fair share of organisms to the microscopic world. Single-cell animals called ***protozoans*** are found in water, foods, blood, and body fluids. Many of these organisms live on plants or rotting tissue; however, some are parasites of people. Amoebic dysentery is caused by a simple, one-cell animal called an amoeba. The severe form of this disease can be fatal. Malaria is caused by a single-cell animal invading the body through a mosquito bite. When the organism enters the bloodstream, the disease can be fatal if not treated properly.

Multiple-cell animals, such as microscopic worms and mites, also cause diseases in people. You should always be looking for lice and scabies. Take special precautions if you see the characteristic bite marks on client's skin. (Figure 2-4.)

FIGURE 2–4
The signs of scabies on skin.

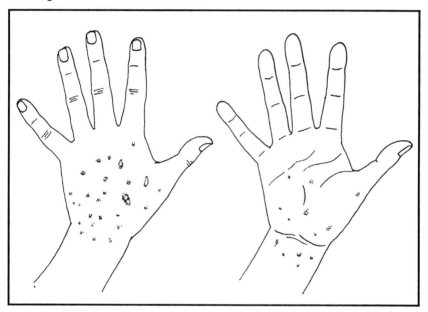

❏ **REVIEW QUESTIONS**

1. What is microbiology?

2. Who is the father of the microscope?

3. What is the purpose of pasteurization?

4. How was the chemical *phenol* used in the 1800s to re-duce the risk of infection caused by the transfer of germs from one person to another?

5. Name the different bacteria classified by shape and give an example of a disease they produce.
6. What is the gram stain technique?
7. Describe the structure of bacteria.
8. Name some examples of fungal infections.
9. List some ways viral particles are spread.

CHAPTER
THREE

Sources of Contamination and Disease

❑ LEARNING OBJECTIVES

After completing this chapter, you should be able to:

- Explain the difference between pathogens and opportunistic microorganisms.

- Identify the sources of contamination that may be present in the salon.

- Discuss the common diseases resulting from exposure to the organisms considered sources of contamination.

- Identify the modes of transmission of microorganisms.

Introduction

In the previous chapters, you learned there is an invisible world of microbes surrounding everything. Most of these microorganisms do not cause any harm. However, there are several types that are capable of infecting people and causing illness. Because these microbes are not visible to the eye, it is easy to forget they can be present in concentration levels high enough to be an infectious risk. This chapter deals with where the sources of infection are found and how infectious agents spread. You need to have an understanding of this in order to effectively develop and use the proper methods of decontamination in the salon.

Chapter Three

Pathogens vs. Opportunistic Microorganisms

A *pathogen* is a microorganism that causes illness in a susceptible person. The only condition required for the pathogen to infect a person is the individual's poor or absent resistance to provide protection from invading microorganisms. This protection is known as *immunity*. Remember, pathogens are disease-producing organisms.

There are other types of microbes not necessarily causing illness. However, if circumstances prevail, and if a person does not have the ability to fight off the microbes, people can be infected by organisms known as *opportunistic microorganisms*. That is, they take advantage of the present opportunity. There are more microbes considered opportunistic than there are pathogens.

Another type of microbe is referred to as the *beneficial microorganism*. These are used, for example, to make bread dough rise (yeast), ferment wine beer and spirits, and to break down organic matter in soil and rotting plants.

In the salon, you should be concerned about the pathogenic and opportunistic microorganisms. All of your clients, and even you and your coworkers, harbor opportunistic microorganisms. These are present in skin, hair, and inside the body. Some of these microorganisms may even be pathogenic since there are people acting as carriers of these microbes. Your clients may never show any symptoms of sickness but can be the sources of transmitting diseases.

When working with the public you should always assume you, your clients, and your co-workers may be carriers of illness. This is why proper infection control techniques must be practiced in your working area, the salon, and not just in hospitals.

Sources of Contamination

Environmental Sources

It is safe to assume you will be exposed to many different microorganisms when working. Some will be pathogenic, and others opportunistic. Certainly you will be exposed to germs causing illness. A germ is a microbe capable of getting a person sick. Germs can be pathogens, or opportunistic microorganisms. In order to adequately protect yourself, your co-workers, and your clients, you must be aware of where these germs are present.

As mentioned, microorganisms are everywhere. They are suspended in the air and are settling constantly on all horizontal surfaces such as countertops, chairs, sinks, and all environmental surfaces in the salon. Germs can hitchhike on the skin, on hair, and on clothing. All these act as primary sources of contamination.

The shampoo sink is notorious for contamination with many different kinds of microorganisms. *Pseudomonas* (a gram negative bacteria) loves warm, moist places, like the sink, whirlpool, soaking bowls, the drain, the water faucet, the cold and hot water controls, and the faucet aerator. The hot and cold water controls, the handles and the tap itself, may be contaminated with the microbes from hands (*staphylococcus* or *streptococcus*), or from someone's hair, nails, or skin.

The implements used during a client's salon visit, like the scissors, files, nippers, and brushes, are other primary sources of contamination. These objects generally contain high levels of organic matter providing ideal growth environments for all microorganisms. Extra precaution must be taken when handling these implements since they are major sources of contamination due to the high level of organic matter they contain.

Microbes may be present in some of the products you are using. For instance, if you have a bar of soap at your shampoo sink or in the bathroom, there is a high probability microbes are growing on the soap. It is well documented that most soaps not only allow germs to survive on soap, but also act as good growth media for some microorganisms. Some lotions, creams, soaking solutions, treatment solutions, and ointments may start out being safe, but over time they lose the preservatives that keep microorganisms from growing. If any of these change color, look unusual, smell musty or develop an unpleasant odor, do not use the product. It may be contaminated with microbes.

Your heating and cooling ventilation systems in the salon may be another source of contamination, especially if the system has not been cleaned and maintained properly. These units have filters and often humidifiers and dehumidifiers. An ideal growth environment is created when filters are not changed and the humidification system is not cleaned. If a mildewy or musty odor is detected, there is a high probability something is growing in the system. Microbes will be blown all over the salon when the blower fan goes on. Legionnaires' disease was spread through the ventilation system of several buildings in a similar manner. Other environmental surfaces such as door handles, chairs, dryers, soaking trays, and tubs are excellent sources of contamination since they, too, come into contact with the single greatest source of microbiologic contamination—people.

The Human Source

People are in constant contact with the environment. We are excellent sources of contamination since we are always shedding dead skin, which has bacteria, fungi, viral particles, and other microorganisms, clinging or feeding on its cells. We have these and other types of microbes living inside our bodies. They are all able to make their way into the environment. When is the last time either you or one of your clients coughed? Occasionally one of your clients will get nicked or cut, and blood might be present. You may get cut, running the risk of being a source of contamination or inviting cross-infection to yourself. (Figure 3–1.)

The United States Occupational Safety and Health Administration (OSHA) has found that blood is a prime source of pathogens (especially the AIDS and hepatitis viruses). OSHA has issued a legal requirement for protecting all healthcare workers, even those only rarely exposed to blood. OSHA calls this the Bloodborne Pathogens Standard. It describes how to prevent being exposed to these pathogens. We might not be exposed to blood often, but the real risk of exposure remains. We must treat any blood contact with extreme caution.

When we touch an object including countertops wall, chairs, or other surfaces, we deposit organic matter and moisture. Some of these contain living microbes. For exam-

FIGURE 3–1
Human contact is the single greatest source of microbiologic contamination. *Photo by Michael A. Gallitelli.*

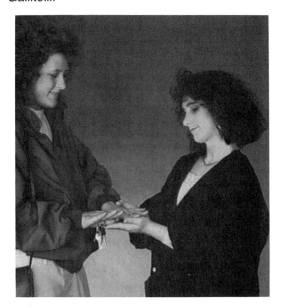

ple, when you touch your face, then grasp a brush with the same hand, brush someone's hair, and set the brush on a countertop, during all those moves you repeatedly deposited organisms. From your face you move microorganisms to your hand; from your hand and the brush it holds you stir up organisms in the client's hair and on the scalp. Some of these are deposited onto the brush and on your hand. In addition, you suspend some dead skin and hair cells in the air along with the microbes present on these surfaces. When you are done using the brush, you deposit falling microbes from the brush and your hand onto the countertop.

So far you have done a good job of contributing to the microflora in the environment. Now let's add to this example. Imagine you and your client are talking. With each breath thousands of droplets of saliva and moisture propel from your bodies. Some, if not all of the droplets, contain microorganisms. Perhaps one of you has a cold, with sneezing and coughing. Colds are caused by virus particles invading the tissues of the respiratory tract. Colds can be spread by either inhaling contaminated droplets in the air, called **airborne transmission**, or by touching a contaminated surface, and then touching your eyes, mouth, or a mucous membrane. This type of transmission is called **indirect transmission** of disease. Simply put, if you touch a contaminated surface and then rub your eyes or lips, you may soon find yourself as sick as your client.

The reality of the situation just described is one of the many ways different germs are spread from one person to another, either through direct contact (kissing, holding hands, and the like) or through indirect contact from a contaminated surface or a dirty implement. Unfortunately, very few people wash their hands between clients or know anything about the hygienic habits of the clients. An estimated 80 percent of the risk of contamination from one person to another comes from either direct or indirect, person-to-person contact. So it really pays to protect yourself by practicing proper infection protection such as cleaning and disinfecting between clients. Very simply, do not forget to wash your hands between clients.

Modes of Transmission of Microorganisms

We have discussed briefly how germs are spread from one person to another. Microorganisms can be spread between people in a variety of modes of transmission. By understanding how germs are transmitted, you will be able to protect yourself and your clients. As you know now, germs can be transferred by direct means such as skin-to-skin contact. If one of your clients is infected with impetigo or ringworm, you would not want to come into contact with the skin because these conditions are extremely contagious. Similarly, you would not want to touch your client's blood or body fluids since there may be infectious agents present.

All of us are aware of how many infections are generally spread through direct contact, especially sexually transmitted diseases. If you have an open cut on your skin and your open cut comes into contact with someone else's blood or body fluid, then there is a real possibility of transferring these agents to yourself without making direct contact with the person. You could infect yourself by touching the blood or fluid left on a pair of scissors or a brush that accidentally nipped the infected client. This method of transmission is another form of indirect transmission.

Another common example of indirect transmission of infectious agents is how easily athlete's foot (a fungus named *trychophyton*) is spread. You do not have to pierce the skin, inhale droplets, or have direct physical contact to spread this germ. If an infected person with athlete's foot walks barefoot on the floor, the infected feet will leave enough sufficient contaminated particles (fungal spores) so the next barefoot person who walks on the same floor might be infected. The fungus will not live forever on the floor, but will remain **viable** (that is, alive) for some time as long as the floor remains warm and moist. If you use a whirlpool or soaking bath in your salon, be sure you thoroughly clean and disinfect these devices with a material that kills the athlete's foot fungus. Also, note many other germs do not need an open path (a cut or a mucous membrane) to infect someone. Yeast infections, scabies, lice, and many skin infections are transmitted this way. If a customer has any kind of skin lesion, be extra careful in your cleaning.

Remember when you were growing up and you were told to wash your hands after going to the bathroom? You were told this for several good reasons. There are some organisms capable of reinfecting people if they do not use good hygiene habits and wash their hands after using the lavatory. Several of these organisms cause food poisoning. One of the principal ways hepatitis A epidemics occur is when a cook (perhaps infected or a carrier) at the local restaurant neglects to wash his or her hands after using the restroom.

Your tools and implements are key instruments you should concentrate on keeping clean and disinfected. Because implements come into contact with the skin, hair, and inanimate surfaces, they are the most ideal means of transmission of microorganisms. Always take special care when handling and decontaminating these objects, for they can be a source of illness for you.

❏ REVIEW QUESTIONS

1. What is the difference between pathogens and opportunistic microorganisms?

2. List some areas in the salon that are the sources of contamination.

3. According to OSHA, what is the prime source of pathogens?

4. How is the common cold caused and spread?

5. Keeping in mind the modes of transmission theory, explain how athlete's foot is spread.

C H A P T E R

F O U R

Breaking the Chain of Cross-Infection

❏ LEARNING OBJECTIVES

After completing this chapter, you should be able to:

- Understand the principles of infection control.

- Explain the differences between cleaning and disinfecting.

- Describe how cleaning agents work.

- Identify the fundamental methods of decontamination.

- Discuss the importance of personal hygiene to reduce the spread of cross-infection.

- Rank the levels of decontamination.

Introduction

Infection control is a combination of basic knowledge of what causes infection, how to control or prevent infection from occurring, and common sense. Proper infection control requires a working understanding of the necessary requisites of the principles of sanitization and personal hygiene. The term *sanitized* implies something is clean and free from germs. This is not true, as you will soon learn. Infection control relies on thorough cleaning and decontaminating.

Cleaning

By definition, ***cleaning*** is the removal of undesirable substances from a surface. This surface can be a living surface, such as skin, or an inanimate object, such as scissors, nippers, chairs, countertops, sinks, walls, floors, and any other object in the salon. Cleaning removes these unwanted substances by utilizing a variety of physical and chemical means. Chemicals that assist cleaning are called ***cleaning agents***. These may be soaps, detergents, wetting agents, shampoos, solvents, and others.

As a general rule, cleaning agents do not kill microorganisms. Cleaning agents merely help in the removal of these microbes from the surfaces requiring cleaning. Dr. Earl Spaulding, a noted professor responsible for the Spaulding Classifications of the levels of decontamination and strengths of microorganisms, observed very early in his career: "You can clean without disinfecting, but you cannot disinfect without cleaning." What Spaulding meant was that you must clean if you are to decontaminate. Cleaning is the first step in the process, but not the entire process.

Cleaning agents are formulated to perform specific functions. For instance, you would not want to wash your hands with a laundry detergent, nor would you shampoo someone's hair with an industrial degreaser. The type of cleaning agent you select determines whether or not you will be successful in your endeavor. The wrong materials for the job may make things worse by creating residues on surfaces, or, even worse, a toxic reaction. Yearly, several people create toxic fumes when they mix household chemicals together trying to make a better cleaner. Do not mix any chemicals together when working with cleaning agents; it can kill you.

How Cleaning Agents Work

Knowing how cleaning agents work will help you choose the right materials to use on the surfaces you need to clean. For example, you would not use a solvent like alcohol on a soft vinyl chair because it would soften the plastic. The pigments used to color the vinyl would wash out and the vinyl might become brittle over time.

Cleaning agents can work several ways:

1. By lifting the soils off the surface and suspending them so they may be rinsed off. This process is called ***emulsification***.

2. By chemically reacting with the soils, particularly the fats that may be present, and then converting the soils to soap. This process is called ***hydrolysis*** or ***saponification***. This is how most soaps are made. Tallow or vegetable oil is reacted with lye to produce natural soap.

3. By dissolving the soils by acting as solvents. On the one hand, most people think of solvents as being organic solvents like alcohol, acetone, or paint remover. Nail polish remover is an organic solvent that is a specialized paint remover. On the other hand, however, the universal solvent is water. Water is a very good solvent. Read the labels on commercial shampoos, creams, soaking agents, and other preparations. You will observe that water is always listed, sometimes as a principal ingredient.

4. By using heat or cold through evaporation or chemical reaction. Heat causes several soils to react with the oxygen in the air. Burning is one of the most obvious forms of cleaning a surface. Temperatures below the ignition point of soils will result in evaporating the soils off the surface. Freezing may free soils stuck on a surface and make the surface clean.

Cleaning agents may incorporate more than one kind of activity in order to work properly. Shampoos have agents that make the dirt and water wetter by breaking down the surface tension between the water molecules. The same shampoo has emulsifying agents to lift the soils off the scalp and hair strands. The water used to dilute the shampoo acts as a solvent, and other solvents may be added to further hasten the cleaning process. This is rather complex.

Soaps vs. Detergents

There is a great difference between soaps and detergents. The only thing they have in common is they both are used to clean things.

Soaps start out as some form of fat. The fat is reacted with lye and other materials are added to the mixture to make it feel better, be less aggressive, or smell good. Chemicals such as glycerin may be added to the soap to provide a silkier, more gentle product. Soaps leave residue. This residue may make the skin feel smoother. Generally, soaps are milder to the skin than detergents because soaps do not remove fat from the skin as much as detergents do.

Detergents are chemically manufactured cleaning agents that function differently than soap. Detergents can break down the surface tension of water and soils, emulsifying and dissolving soils; but they cannot convert fatty soils into soap. Detergents are generally free rinsing; that is, when you rinse them, little or no residue is left behind. Many detergents do not require rinsing at all. However, detergents are much more aggressive to the skin and soils than soaps are. So, more care should be exercised when using them than when using soaps.

Disinfection, Sanitization, and Sterilization

Once cleaning has been accomplished, the more difficult part of the decontamination process needs to be done. Typically, this includes killing germs. In the salon, your attention should be focused on disinfection. **Disinfection** is the process of killing specific microorganisms by any physical or chemical means. Most people are familiar with the chemical means of disinfection. There are several levels of disinfection as described by Spaulding. These levels are based on the ability to kill organisms that have increasing resistance to the chemical disinfectant. There are four levels of disinfection efficacy:

1. limited disinfection (very low level)
2. general disinfection (low level)
3. hospital-grade disinfection (plain)
4. hospital-grade *tuberculocidal* disinfection (ideal).

A limited-efficacy, low-level disinfectant will not kill the organism causing tuberculosis (TB). It will not kill *pseudomonas*, the marker-organism for hospital-grade disinfectants. (See chapter 8.) Most household disinfectants, as limited-efficacy products (very low level) will kill either *staphylococcus* or *salmonella*, but not both. Low-level disinfection is not broad-spectrum disinfection. Even though low-level disinfectants can kill either gram positive or gram negative organisms, they cannot kill both.

General disinfectants (low level) will not kill the TB organis, or *pseudomonas*; however, they will kill both *staphylococcus* and *salmonella* (gram positive and gram negative organisms, respectively). This is why a hospital-level disinfectant is better than a general one, but is still not ideal.

Hospital-grade disinfection involves killing *staphylococcus*; *salmonella*, and *pseudomonas aeruginosa*, which is a more difficult bacteria to kill than many viruses. Hospital-grade disinfection does not kill *mycobacteria tuberculosis*.

The TB organism has a hard, waxy, outer coating acting as a shield, preventing lower-level disinfectants from harming it. The ability to kill the TB bacillus with a hospital-grade (plain) disinfectant is the distinguishing characteristic between a hospital-grade disinfectant and the ideal, hospital-grade tuberculocidal disinfectant. The ideal choice for today's salon infection control is a tuberculocidal, hospital-grade disinfectant. Interestingly, however, tuberculosis is not communicable from an environmental surface in most cases, yet new cases of blood-to-blood transmission have been reported. The benefits of hospital-level tuberculocidal disinfection include:

1. It is the ideal level of disinfection available.

2. It is a broad-spectrum disinfectant suitable for the salon infection control.

3. It kills TB, which has a very hard outer coat that is more difficult to penetrate than *pseudomonas*.

Therefore, when a disinfectant is able to kill TB, as hospital-level tuberculocidal disinfection does, it offers the ideal degree of broad-spectrum efficacy (germ-killing ability). Broad spectrum means it is active against a wide variety of microorganisms including staph, salmonella, pseudomonas, some fungal and viral particles. OSHA prefers hospital-grade tuberculocidal disinfection for salon infection control. Remember, disinfecting is not the same as sterilizing, nor as sanitization.

Why is the tuberculosis organism used as an indicator of a disinfectant's efficacy? It is used as a marker organism for killing more resistant strains of microbes. The *tuberculosis bacillus* is considered one of the most difficult organisms to kill due to its increased resistance. If a disinfectant can kill TB, the same disinfectant will be able to kill many of the more resistant organisms.

Sterilization differs from disinfection in many ways. First, sterilization kills all forms of biologic life, including the bacterial spore. Some bacteria, but not all, produce spores when the conditions for survival no longer exist. Bacterial spores are the most resistant forms of life on earth. A bacterial spore is up to 10,000 times more resistant to disinfectants than when it is in its active, growing form. Sterilization kills bacterial spores, whereas disinfection does not.

Second, sterilization is generally accomplished by using a sterilizing chamber, such as a steam autoclave, which rises the temperature and pressure so high that all life is destroyed. Other methods of sterilization include the use of ethylene oxide gas in a chamber, or extremely dangerous chemicals that should be handled under a chemical fume hood by experts. Remember, these materials kill everything and are extremely hazardous. The salon should not smell of formaldehyde or glutaraldehyde. Both are toxic chemicals. If the salon smelled of these chemicals, you would not have clients. The odor, coupled with burning eyes and noses, would keep them away. Disinfection is a method of choice for decontaminating the salon when compared to sterilization. It is impossible to sterilize a salon without destroying it, but it is very practical to disinfect almost everything in the salon.

Another common term that is misused is sanitization. In the health and beauty industries, many professionals refer to the degerming process of sanitizing. Sanitizing is a process that removes the bulk of easy-to-kill microorganisms from a previously cleaned surface. It is inefficient, wasteful of time, money, and supplies. Sanitizing requires you first wash the surface with a cleaner, rinse with water, and then apply an agent that does not kill 100 percent of the microbes. Those microbes that survive are usually the more resistant forms of the same strains, and because they are stronger they may be the source of contamination and disease. Why bother sanitizing when all the microbes can be killed with a disinfectant?

To summarize, sterilization is not practical in a salon. A room cannot be sterilized. If you want to sterilize equipment, cleaning and disinfecting will render them safe to handle before sterilizing anyway. Sanitizing is not a method of choice in the salon either. Sanitizing does not kill the organism completely and is wasteful of supplies and labor. Disinfection is the method that should be used to effectively decontaminate the salon setting, killing the germs without creating a hostile environment for you and the clients. Because of the increasing risk of exposure to infectious agents, you should set your disinfection standards only to intermediate-level disinfection. This level will provide the ideal degree of protection.

The one and only level of infection control for the salon is broad-spectrum hospital-grade, *tuberculocidal disinfection*.

Personal Hygiene

Personal hygiene should not be overlooked when developing a plan to keep the salon free from risk of exposure to infectious agents. The most important step you and your co-workers can take to reduce the spread of cross-infection is to wash your hands. Always wash your hands between clients, after touching your face, mouth, or other body parts, after providing any service, and after using and handling implements. An FDA-listed, antimicrobial liquid hand soap with an NDC number on its label is suggested for hand disinfection. If the liquid soap is made of cosmetic-grade ingredients, it will be less irritating to skin. Cosmetic-grade chemicals have fewer impurities, which are the sources of irritants. If the soap contains emollients (skin-conditioning agents), or is lotion-based, it will be less likely to dry your skin out. An antimicrobial soap that kills germs is best to use.

Skincare lotions, protective skin creams, and similar kinds of products should be applied before lunch, breaks, and at the end of the work day. It is not a good idea to use these products between clients because they may act as magnets which attract and hold microbes on the skin. In addition, they may leave a fine residue that is difficult to remove on the handles of the brushes and implements. Finally, this coating will become excellent growth media for microbes, breeding germs and opportunistic microorganisms rather than removing them.

Levels of Decontamination

There are several levels of decontamination available. Table 4–1 shows their ranking.

TABLE 4–1: Levels of Decontamination

Sterilized
Hospital-grade tuberculocidal ideal-efficacy disinfected
High-level, intermediate-efficacy disinfected
General, low-level efficacy disinfected
Limited, low-level disinfected
Sanitized
Visually clean
Moderately clean (residues present)
Swept
Contaminated

❑ **REVIEW QUESTIONS**

1. What is infection control?

2. What is cleaning?

3. Describe emulsification in respect to working with cleaning agents.

4. How are most soaps made?

5. What are the differences between soaps and detergents?

6. What are the four levels of disinfection efficacy?

7. What are the benefits of hospital-level tuberculocidal disinfection?

8. How does sterilization differ from disinfection?

9. How is sterilization generally accomplished?

10. Why is disinfection the method of choice for decontaminating the salon when compared to sterilization?

11. What is the process of sanitizing? Why is sanitizing inefficient in the salon?

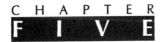

C H A P T E R
FIVE

Decontaminating Materials and Procedures

❏ **LEARNING OBJECTIVES**

After completing this chapter, you should be able to:

■ Explain the differences between one-step and two-step germicidal cleaners.

■ List the active ingredients used to disinfect.

■ Decide what kinds of decontaminating agents would be appropriate for use in the salon.

■ Identify the attributes necessary for products to decontaminate the salon environment and the general conditions for use.

■ Discuss phenolic compounds, quaternary ammonium compounds, iodophor-based disinfectants, alcohols, and hypochlorites and list their advantages and limitations.

■ List the factors affecting the performance of disinfectants.

Introduction

Not all decontaminating materials are made of the same materials nor do they work in the same way. As you learned in the earlier chapters, cleaners work in a variety of ways. Decontaminating agents, specifically, the disinfecting agents, can also work in different ways depending upon their formulation and their intended uses.

One-Step vs. Two-Step Germicidal Cleaners

Some disinfecting agents are formulated to clean, disinfect, and deodorize simultaneously. These are called one-step germicidal cleaners. Their formulas contain cleaning agents compatible with germ-killing agents. Making a formula to do both jobs is rather complicated. If the wrong detergent or soap is used, it will cancel out the germ-killing abilities of the product. You should never mix chemicals.

Most of the chemicals from the supermarket are not strong enough to kill germs properly. Those household products having good disinfecting properties have to be used at concentration levels creating potentially toxic fumes and might be corrosive to the surfaces they are used on. Household bleach is an example of this type of compound. To get the full benefits of bleach's germ-killing abilities, you need to use a strength of one part bleach to ten to one hundred parts of water. This concentration will kill the germs but will also damage most surfaces including your tools and implements. Never soak instruments in bleach; bleach will destroy them. Bleach will soften nylon combs. Bleach is not a cleaning agent. Most people are sensitive to the swimming pool odor that bleach gives off. This is a form of chlorine that can be toxic if the concentration levels of the fumes get high enough.

Bleach is a good example of a two-step disinfectant. You must clean the surface with a cleaning agent, rinse, and apply bleach to the surface. Using two-step products like bleach is rather impractical because it is costly and labor intensive. The newer one-step germicidal cleaners (disinfectant cleaners) are much more efficient and may actually cost less to use.

Types of Disinfectants

There are many possible active ingredients used to kill microorganisms. The active ingredients used to disinfect are listed in Table 5-1.

TABLE 5–1: Disinfectants

A. *Chemical Disinfectants*

Liquids and Gases

Phenols, phenates	Hydrogen peroxide
Quaternary ammonium compounds	Mineral acids
	Organic acids
Idophors, Iodine-based compounds	Steam
	B-propiolactone
Alcohols: ethanol, isopropal, combinations, cetyl	Mercurials
	Silver salts
Chlorine-containing compounds: hypochlorites, chlorine dioxide, chloramine	Ozone
	Chlorhexidine
Aldehydes: formaldehyde, glutaraldehyde	Peracetic acid
	ETO
Plasma/vapor base	Other salts: copper, sulphur, bromine, caustic soda

B. *Physical Disinfectants*

Dry heat	Differential pressure	Ultraviolet light
Microwave	New methods	

Many of these chemicals are exotic and not used very often. You would not want to use a silver salt on countertops or chairs because the silver salts will leave a black, streaky residue considered a contaminant itself. Nor would you use a strong inorganic acid such as hydrochloric or sulfuric acid. These materials not only will clean and kill germs, but also they react with surfaces and dissolve them. Sulfuric acid is an ingredient in some drain openers and is extremely hazardous to handle. Hydrochloric acid is one of the most aggressive compounds available. When it reacts with some surfaces, a major toxic by-product (chlorine gas) is produced. It is hazardous if inhaled for more than a few breaths.

Selecting the appropriate cleaner and disinfectant for the salon is not easy. You are not expected to be a chemist or microbiologist. To ease your decisions, several excellent, commercially available compounds are available. Most of these compounds do not use strong mineral acids or exotic heavy metal in their formulas. Only a few of the *active ingredients* (the materials killing germs) are used to formulate commercially available one-step and two-step disinfection products. They are:

1. Phenols or phenolics
2. Quaternary ammonium compounds (quats)
3. Alcohol or alcohol based
4. Bleach or hypochlorite
5. Iodine or iodophor based
6. Pine oil based
7. Mild acids, such as vinegar

Each of these materials has its own advantages and disadvantages. However, some are much better than others, and some hardly work at all. When selecting a germicidal cleaner for the salon, you should use materials that are marginally acceptable because the people you could place in an exposed environment include yourself. So why risk getting sick?

Active Ingredients: Advantages and Disadvantages

Home-Use Disinfectants

Most salon operators still think supermarket or home-use disinfectants are strong enough for the salon. Household-strength disinfecting agents do not have the strength to kill a wide variety of germs in the salon environment, especially with the volume of people coming into the salon on a daily basis. Most of the materials sold in the retail market (grocery stores, drug stores, discount stores, and the like) lack the concentration of active ingredients necessary to kill a wide variety of gram positive and gram negative bacteria, *pseudomonas*, and the *tuberculosis bacillus*.

Minimum Disinfectant Requirements

The first criteria in selecting a disinfectant cleaner or germicidal cleaner is that it kills these bacteria. The germicidal cleaner should at least be effective against *staphylococcus aureus, salmonella choleraesius*, and *pseudomonas aeruginosa*. This is the same criteria the Environmental Protection Agency (EPA) uses to determine the disinfecting agent classification when a germicide's product-formula is registered. The EPA is the governmental regulating agency responsible for disinfectants, sterilants, and sanitizing agents. Biocidal efficacy (the ability to kill specific organisms) is one of the key points used by the EPA to classify the strength of these agents. Household products, not able to kill all three basic bacteria indicated, are classified as weaker than those products killing these bacteria. Agents killing the TB bacteria are considered yet stronger than those not able to kill TB.

Biocidal efficacy (the ability to kill the organisms) against TB is essential if there is any likelihood of the presence of blood or body fluids. The germicidal cleaner should also demonstrate efficacy against fungi (*trychophyton*) and some viruses such as the flu virus (*influenza*), herpes virus, and the AIDS virus.

Phenolic-Based Disinfectants

The phenolic-based disinfectant formulas usually have many of these characteristics, for this reason, the formulas using the phenolics as active ingredients are usually preferred. Phenolic-based chemicals are excellent, since they have very few limitations.

Phenols were originally discovered in the mid-1800s by Dr. Joseph Lister, a surgeon deeply concerned about most patients dying from undergoing surgery from either blood poisoning or infection. Even though the germ theory was not fully described, Lister set out to find ways to reduce the mortality rate from surgery. In one of his experiments, Lister stilled a compound from coal tar. The compound was a crude phenol: carbolic acid. Lister washed his hands in this material before operating, washed his surgical instruments, and washed the operating table, and even made surgical dressings soaked in the material for use on patients after surgery. Surprisingly, many of Lister's patients, who would have previously died if not for the phenolic compound's effects survived the surgery. The advantages of phenolic compounds follow:

1. Phenols have an extremely broad range of germ-killing activity including *tuberculosis bacillus* and quite a few other resistant microbes. This type of activity is referred to as **broad-spectrum efficacy**.

2. Phenolics are not affected generally by organic matter as much as other compounds.

3. Phenolics have a proven use history. When buffered, they are safer to humans and the environment than other disinfectants.

Phenolic compounds have some limitations. They include:

1. If the wrong type of cleaning agent is mixed with the phenolic active ingredients, the effectiveness of the

phenols may be reduced or destroyed. Phenolic-based germicidal cleaners have to be developed very carefully, and should not be mixed with any detergents or other chemicals.

2. Some phenolic disinfecting agents have a medicinal or hospital-like smell to them. Smell or fragrance is very subjective. You might like the smell of roses and someone else may be offended by it. Germicidal cleaning agents are formulated to kill the odor-causing bacteria not to smell good. If they were formulated to smell good, you might be apt to overuse these products and create an unsafe, toxic environment as a result.

3. Some phenolic compounds can cause rubber and some plastics to swell if soaked in the phenolic solution for a long period of time. As with all disinfecting agents, there must be sufficient contact time with the germs for proper efficacy to transpire. This contact time is called ***dwell time*** and is always specified on the product's label. Reading and interpreting product labels are discussed in the next chapter.

4. Some phenolic-based germicides can make the skin feel like it is burning when gloves are not worn. This is an excellent warning mechanism that tells the user to always wear gloves when using these or any disinfecting agents. Most other disinfecting agents do not produce a tingling sensation when in contact with the skin. They just produce a chemical burn after exposure. The phenolic-based germicidal agents provide this advanced warning mechanism, thus preventing this kind of burn if the warning is heeded. (This is an important advantage of the phenols.)

Quaternary Ammonium Compounds

Quaternary ammonium compounds are chloride based disinfecting agents. Quats, as they are commonly called, have been present since the early part of this century (1919–1920). Quats are found in many laundry detergents, cleaning agents, and are present in many skin preparations as preservatives, as well as cleaning agents. A preservative keeps microorganisms from growing in a product. These compounds are synthetically produced wetting agents. They actually make surfaces "wetter" by breaking down the surface tension of materials with which they come in contact. In an earlier chapter, you learned that water was the universal solvent. When a drop of water is placed on a smooth surface, it forms a bead. When a quat is mixed with the water it will not bead up but rather it will become a thin film. This is the action of the quat—the wetting agent, also called the **surfactant**. Quats use this characteristic to their advantage as disinfecting agents by acting on the cell wall of the microbe. The surfactant activity of the quat in contact with fats that are present on the cell wall of the microbe results in these fats breaking down. This causes microscopic "holes" in the cell wall, which allow the fluids inside the cell to escape causing death. The scientific term for this action is called **lysis** (of the cell). Unfortunately, quats lack the strength necessary to penetrate the *tuberculosis bacillus* outer shell and do not cause lysis to occur in this organism.

The advantages of quats include the following:

1. Excellent cleaning agents and are very compatible with many other wetting agents.

2. Quats contain excellent disinfecting properties against gram positive bacteria and are very effective on easy-to-kill bacteria.

3. Quats are relatively non-toxic in solution.

4. Quats may be used on food preparation surfaces. (Some do not require rinsing at all.)

5. Quats contain excellent deodorizing properties. They can be blended with fragrances easily, thus providing an acceptable smell.

The disadvantages of quats include the following:

1. Quats are inactive against tuberculosis and other resis-

tant organisms, including some viruses.

2. Quats are sensitive to the minerals in tap water and moderate amounts of organic matter (blood). Quats may be inactivated by hard water, not distilled water, and there minerals will be present. These minerals act as magnets and latch onto the quat molecules, thus rapidly consuming the active ingredients. Blood and other forms of organic matter act just like the hard water minerals, seeking out the actives and inactivating them. If you are going to use a quaternary ammonium chloride-based disinfecting system, always check on the label to make sure it is effective in hard water and in 5 percent blood serum. This will at least give you some assurance that the product you selected will work in the "real" world and not just in a research laboratory.

3. Quats may cause staining and discoloration of metal surfaces if improperly used.

4. Quats have a "fishy" smell without fragrances.

Iodophors and Iodine-Based Disinfectants

You might remember getting cut or scraped and putting a tincture of iodine on the injury. The cut would sting and be uncomfortable. The skin would become stained. Iodine is used as a skin antiseptic, preventing infection. The use of iodine as a wound antiseptic is traced back to the mid-1800s. Dr. Robert Koch was a scientist who worked with microbiology. He set the foundation for many of today's methods. Koch used iodine to inactivate anthrax spores, demonstrating iodine's disinfecting abilities. Advances and refinements in creating easier-to-use forms of iodine resulted in the discovery of the ***iodophors***, the modern version of iodine.

Iodophor-based disinfecting agents are very effective in many applications because they have good disinfecting properties. However, there are significant drawbacks precluding the use of these formulas in the salon, the last of which is the difficulty in handling.

Advantages of iodophor-based disinfectants include:

1. Iodophors are very effective against some viruses and are excellent against the gram positive and some gram negative bacteria.

2. Some iodophor-based formulas are used to sanitize food contact surfaces.

3. Iodophor-based formulas may be used to disinfect drinking water.

4. Iodophors have very quick microbial killing times.

Unfortunately, the disadvantages outweigh the benefits of these compounds. The disadvantages include:

1. Iodine-based disinfecting agents are not good cleaners. Remember, cleaning must precede disinfecting.

2. Iodine-based disinfecting compounds, when used on environmental surfaces (e.g., floors, walls, client chairs, countertops) will stain them all a golden yellow color. The stain will be either difficult or impossible to remove. Even the most modern iodophor-based disinfectant exhibits this staining characteristic. The stain is unsightly and makes the surfaces appear as if they are soiled or dirty even though they are clean. A cardinal rule in salon conditions is that a clean-looking salon helps your clients feel comfortable, and thus, satisfied with the results.

3. Iodine-based compounds are readily inactivated by ultraviolet light. The primary sources of ultraviolet light are sunlight, artificial sunlight from tanning beds, sun lamps, and the fluorescent lights used in many salons as the main source of light. Some nail-hardening treatments rely on the use of an ultraviolet curing light, which would inactivate this disinfectant, too. Now you know why tincture of iodine is sold in a dark brown bottle rather than clear glass.

4. Iodine-based products are extremely sensitive to exposure to organic materials. Even minor amounts of or-

ganic matter will use up the available iodine and render it ineffective.

5. Iodine-based disinfectants are equally sensitive to hard water minerals. This is why iodine-based disinfectants can be used to treat drinking water. They get used up rapidly with little risk of consuming them in the water.

6. If a microorganism happens to survive in a weak solution of iodophors, there is a risk of developing an iodine-resistant strain of that microorganism. This is what happened in the 1980s in Illinois. A manufacturer of these iodophors for use in hospitals neglected to treat the water being used when making the compounds. *Pseudomonas* was present in the water and thus was introduced into the product that was supposed to kill it. *Pseudomonas* (a gram negative bacteria) survived and developed into a strain resistant to specific iodophors. The Food and Drug Administration (FDA) took action and removed the product from the market. It was later learned that even some disinfecting agents will support the growth of the very microbes they are supposed to kill. This is another reason why iodophors and iodine-based disinfecting agents are not recommended for use. In addition, they can have offensive odors.

Alcohols as Disinfecting Agents

Throughout recorded history, alcohol, in various forms, has been used as a disinfecting agent, a skin disinfectant, and a sanitizing agent. One common misconception is that alcohols sterilize. They are not sterilants.

Although alcohol is tuberculocidal, it is a very poor disinfectant and does not kill flu-like viruses. Added to this, alcohol is weakened easily by organic matter. Also, notice alcohol is expensive since it is a two-step process; first, you must clean (alcohol does not clean); second, you must disinfect. Importantly, alcohol is flammable and a fire hazard to use. Lastly, alcohol is pH sensitive. (See the discussion on pH later in this chapter.)

The Hypochlorites (Bleach)

Bleach is an excellent disinfecting agent. Commercial bleaches (from the supermarket) are 5.25 percent sodium or potassium hypochlorite solutions in water, a somewhat strong solution. Owing to their strength, these common bleach formulas can whiten clothing. Household bleach requires surfaces to be thoroughly cleaned before disinfection because bleach is a very poor cleaning agent. Even the new formulas on the market containing cleaning agents do not do good jobs of cleaning, so precleaning is always necessary.

Bleach is a two-step, labor-intensive disinfecting agent. A one-to-ten (one part bleach to ten parts water) to a one–to–one-hundred concentration is required to achieve broad-spectrum disinfection. Bleach releases noxious fumes, similar to the smell of swimming pools; these fumes can cause respiratory distress.

Never mix bleach with any other cleaning or disinfecting agent (or any chemical for that matter). The result could be disastrous or even fatal. A form of nerve gas is made by mixing bleach, vinegar, and TSP (the cleaning agent found in many household cleaners. When used by itself, TSP is effective. Beware that a mixture of bleach and TSP can be fatal.

Another harmful combination is bleach with acids. Never use bleach on metal since bleach will pit the metal and cause corrosion (rust). Additionally, the sharp edges of metal instruments will dull and produce reactions between the metal and the bleach forming deposits on the instruments.

Factors Affecting the Performance of Disinfectants

There are seven factors affecting how a disinfectant system will work in your salon:

1. dilution of the disinfection solution

2. contact time of objects in the solution (dwell time)

3. water (tap water and hard minerals)

4. types of soils to be removed from objects
   to be disinfected

5. pH

6. temperature

7. you

There are essentially only two types of products used to clean, disinfect, or do both simultaneously. They are concentrated formulas (requiring mixing) and ready-to-use formulas (premixed). Both of these types of formulas have advantages and disadvantages.

Concentrated products are generally more economical to use since they are mixed with water by the end-user, not shipped premixed with water by the manufacturer. Of course, premixed products cost the end-user more money in shipping and in having the manufacturer add the water to it. Additionally, ready-to-use products require stabilizers to keep them ready to use, contributing to cost.

Concentrated products require proper measuring and mixing to ensure the use solution (the mixed solution) will work as specified on the label of the product. People often assume the more product, the better it will work. This is untrue when it comes to disinfecting agents since the killing power of these agents is specifically focused to work at the dilution level indicated on the product label. (Figure 5–1.) Too much or too little could mean the product will not do anything. Too much produces either a milky white solution in the mixing container, or a milky white residue on the bottom of the mixing container.

Some cleaners work better when a greater amount than recommended is used. However, removing the residue from these cleaners becomes difficult. Too much is not good and too little is no good. Always follow label directions.

There are products available with premeasured pumps, unit-dose (premeasured) packets or pouches, eliminating

FIGURE 5–1
Dilution and disinfectant activity.

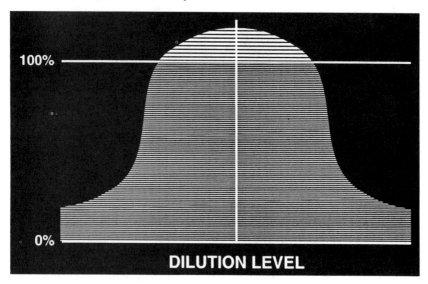

the possibility of mixing incorrectly, costing about the same as very large containers when compared with the actual use-cost of the products.

Again, ready-to-use products take the guess work out of mixing, but they cost much more to use. These products limit the user's ability to have new, fresh solution when and where it is needed.

Contact Time

Time is one of the most important factors when disinfecting. There is a certain amount of time necessary for a product to perform to 100 percent of its label claims. By not following label directions and by disregarding the contact time indicated on the product label, one breaks federal law. Always provide the contact time as specified on the product label.

You may have used a cleaning agent you felt did not work well. Chances are you did not allow sufficient time for the cleaning agent to penetrate and lift the soil.

Allow time for disinfection to happen, or you could create resistant forms of microorganisms. A two-second wipe with a product is not disinfection. Use full-immersion, broad-spectrum, hospital-grade, tuberculocidal disinfectants, which take only ten minutes. (Figure 5–2.)

FIGURE 5–2
Time is one of the most important factors when disinfecting.

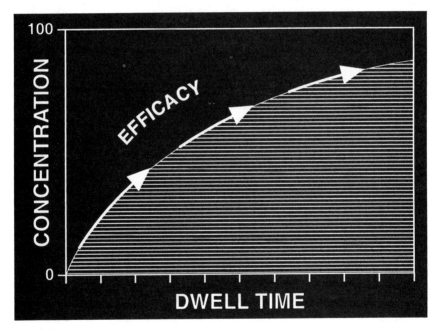

Water (The Universal Solvent or Our Universal Problem?)

Concentrated germicidal cleaners, all-purpose cleaners, and disinfecting agents are all diluted with tap water. The quality of tap water can range from very soft (like New York City) to very hard (like Hartford, Wisconsin). Minerals in the water govern the quality of the water in relation to disinfectant products. These minerals in the water can even in-activate disinfecting solutions. A disinfecting agent is only as good as the water it is in. If the water is hard water (over 60 parts per million [ppm] of hardness), then one should use a hard-water-effective germicidal cleanser. Hard water leaves a white ring or film on surfaces.

New York City has soft water (around 30 ppm). One can tell when the water is soft when it takes longer to rinse surfaces after cleaning. Cleaning solutions will feel soapy, with a silky-slick feeling on clean surfaces in soft water areas. However, outside of places like New York City, water is ob-tained from wells providing very hard water (200 ppm).

Water from the Great Lakes is very hard. Hartford, Wiscon-sin, a suburb of Milwaukee, has very hard water (around 760 ppm). This level of hardness must be softened for dis-infectants and cleaning agents to work. People should find out their water hardness by contacting the local water com-pany or local utilities board. This information will be help-ful in determining whether you need to install a water softener. Softened water makes cleaning skin, hair, and all inanimate objects easier, providing excellent results. (See charts on pages 55 and 56.)

Types of Soils

The type of soil to be removed affects how a cleaning agent or disinfectant works. Organic soils (such as blood, hair, nails, clippings, body fat, makeup, soaps, and skin condi-tioners) are normally organic compounds. Some disinfect-ing agents are inactivated in the presence of even small amounts of organic matter. Iodine-based compounds, alco-hol, and bleach are affected dramatically by organic matter. Also, quats are affected by organic matter. Be sure if you are using a quat the label states it is effective in 5 percent blood serum, a better quat solution able to withstand more organ-ic matter.

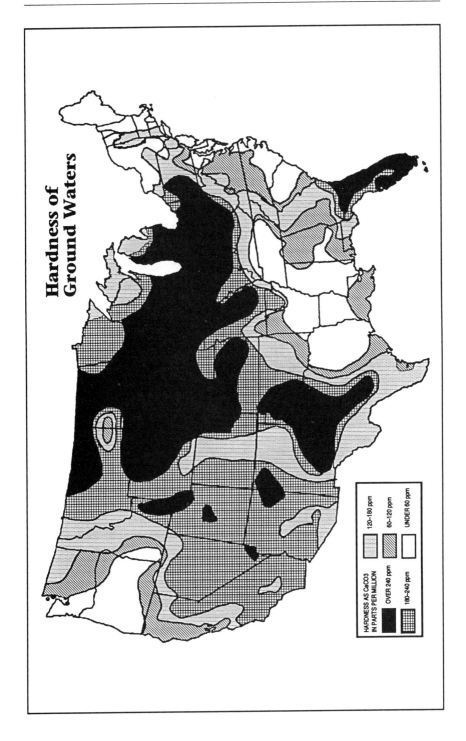

Hardness of Ground Waters

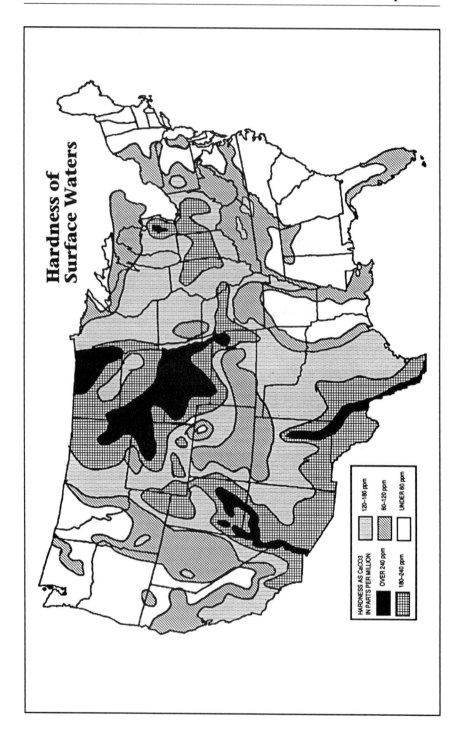

Hardness of
Surface Waters

HARDNESS AS CaCO3
IN PARTS PER MILLION

OVER 240 ppm

180–240 ppm

120–180 ppm

60–120 ppm

UNDER 60 ppm

Because many of the products used in salons (e.g., creams, lotions) as well as hair, nails, are organic in nature, it is important you select either a 5 percent blood-serum-effective disinfecting agent or a tuberculocidal one. The optimum level of disinfection for the salon is a tuberculocidal disinfectant. (Figure 5–3.)

FIGURE 5–3
Germicidal cleaning.

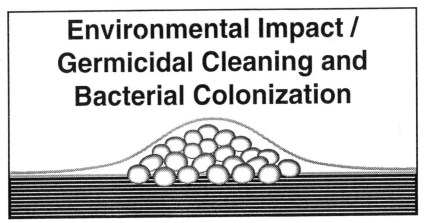

pH

pH is perhaps the most misunderstood chemical term. pH is nothing more than a scale of measurement of the degree of acidity (acid nature) or alkalinity (basic nature) as compared to pure water (untreated water containing no minerals). Every object has a pH.

The pH scale ranges from 0 to 14. At the center of the scale is 7 (neutral). Neutral means it is neither acid or alkaline. Pure water is neutral and has a pH value of 7.

Acids are materials with a pH value below 7. The farther away from 7 and toward 0, the more acidic the material. For example, human skin is around 5.5. Vinegar is around 4 and is, therefore, more acidic than skin because it is farther down the scale and closer to 0.

Hydrochloric acid and sulfuric acid have very low pH levels (around 1–2) and are very aggressive chemicals because of their degrees of acidity. For this reason, one would not want to use them to disinfect surfaces or instruments since they could damage them due to their strong acidic nature.

Any material having a pH above 7 is referred to as alkaline or basic. Examples of alkaline materials are blood (pH 7), milk (pH 10 approximately), and lye (pH 14 approximately). The farther away from 7 a material is, the stronger it is. Many of the most aggressive cleaning agents, like the ones used to clean clothing (laundry detergents), surfaces (cleansers and detergents), hair, and nails (soaps and shampoos) are alkaline.

The relationship between pH and disinfection is a critical one. Disinfectants need to work in the real world, not merely in laboratory tests. Here one must pay particular attention to pH. Be aware of the use-dilution (the pH of the product after dilution) when choosing a salon disinfectant. All microorganisms we do not want to be in contact with have a specified pH range of survival. This survival pH range is between 3.9 and 9.5. Germs can grow and reproduce within this pH range. Note each type of microorganism has a different pH range for its survival. For example, the pH of athlete's foot fungus is around 4.0–6.8. *Pseudomonas* can survive throughout the entire range of 3.9–9.5, but mostly prefers the alkaline range (7.1–9.5). When choosing a disinfectant, one should choose one maintaining a pH range outside of this growth and survival range of 3.5–9.5. By choosing a disinfectant outside of this range, a hostile environment for microorganisms is present and thus the risk of spreading disease is greatly reduced.

Another advantage of using a disinfectant outside of this range of growth and reproduction (3.5–9.5) is the issue of safety. When a hostile environment is set up to keep these organisms from growing, the manufacturer can use less of the killing agents commonly called biocides, and thus there is less exposure to these biocides because less is being used to achieve the same result. The net result is a much safer product to use.

The ideal pH range for germicidal cleaning agents and or disinfectants is between 2.6 and 3.2 on the acid side of the pH scale and between 10 and 11 on the alkaline side of the ph scale. A pH range of below 2.6 or above 11 would result in chemicals that would certainly kill the germs but would also be harmful to the user and the surfaces being treated. Remember to always check the use-dilution of the products you are considering, and not the concentrate dilution. These will have a different pH. Additionally, a pH in the 2.6–3.2 and 10–11 ranges allows a disinfection product to last longer, continuing to work. Mix first, then measure the pH to get an accurate reading of how the product will behave in a real-life situation (in a salon, day to day). (Figure 5–4.)

FIGURE 5–4
Disinfectants, pathogens, and pH.

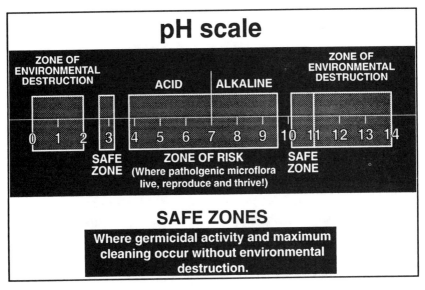

Temperature

Temperature can have an effect on a cleaning agent's removal of certain soils. A hot solution might work better than a cold solution because the heat allows the solution to penetrate faster and remove the soils more easily. This is only true with cleansers and not disinfectants.

Disinfectants should be used at room temperature or with cold water. EPA-registered disinfectants and germicidal cleaners work at room temperature. Should the temperature be elevated, there is no difference in how well the product will kill microorganisms, but what could result are unpleasant vapors from the solution causing bad smells and respiratory distress.

Corrosion

An important factor in selecting a disinfectant is whether or not it will cause corrosion to the object to be treated. The most common form of corrosion is rust. Rust is caused by the reaction of the oxygen present in the water used in diluting the disinfecting product and the iron-based metals in the instruments being treated with the solution. It is possible to cause stainless steel to rust. Always choose a disinfectant that contains a rust inhibitor.

Should one be using chrome-plated equipment, you may notice the surfaces look dull after using the disinfectant or cleaner. This is a form of corrosion. Chrome-plated instruments with sharp edges become blunt or dull should corrosion begin to occur. It is also likely if people leave a pool of disinfectant or cleaning agents around the legs of chairs and tables, the same dulling effect would take place.

Often black gummy residues are confused with corrosion or rust. The gummy residues are merely the build up of dirt, creams, lotions, gels, and acrylics on the instruments and can be removed easily with steel wool, acetone or steel wool and acetone. Corrosion is pitting, dulling, or the actual change of color to a metal surface.

The residues corrosion form are not harmful themselves but are unsightly to clients and provide an ideal environment for microorganisms to grow and reproduce.

Always make sure you use products not causing corrosion. If the label of the product does not mention anything about corrosion, contact the manufacturer and ask if it does. Why destroy equipment unnecessarily?

You

You are the most important part of the cleaning and disinfecting process. You choose the materials to be used for disinfection and cleaning. You decide how they are to be used (hopefully by reading labels and following instructions), and finally you apply these materials. Even though manufacturers can create superior formulas, these disinfecting and cleaning products work only when used properly and according to directions. Also, all of these materials require some old-fashioned elbow grease when using them. Do not be afraid to scrub gently if the surface is dirty, or should you want to save some effort, allow the material to soak for some time before scrubbing. Allow the chemicals sufficient time to work. Your eyes will deceive you. Gross soils and dirt are visible, but microorganisms are not. Do not assume because there are no visible soils that there are no germs.

You can and do make the difference when it comes to disinfection and personal protection.

❏ REVIEW QUESTIONS

1. What is the difference between one-step and two-step germicidal cleaners?

2. Name the active ingredients used to formulate commercially available one-step and two-step disinfection products.

3. What is the EPA?

4. What is the criteria the EPA uses to determine the classification of a disinfecting agent when a germicide's product formula is registered?

5. What is biocidal efficacy?

6. List some advantages of phenolic compounds.

7. List some advantages of quats.

8. List some advantages of iodophor-based disinfectants.

9. Why is alcohol a poor disinfectant?

10. Why should bleach never be mixed with any other cleaning or disinfecting agent?

11. Name the seven factors affecting how a disinfectant will work in the salon.

12. What determines the hardness or softness of water? What is preferred for effective cleaning?

13. What is the ideal pH range for germicidal cleaning agents and/or disinfectants?

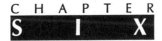

Sterilization

❏ **LEARNING OBJECTIVES**

After completing this chapter, you should be able to:

■ Define sterilization.

■ Understand the principles of sterilization and the methods available for use.

■ Recognize the limits to sterilization.

■ Discuss the place of sterilization in the salon.

Introduction

Sterilization is the destruction of all forms of microbiological life forms. When an object is sterilized, nothing remains alive. Most people think of sterilization as a process confined to hospitals and surgeons' medical instruments. Practically speaking, these are accurate observations since in our day-to-day lives sterilization is not always necessary. Sterilization is appropriate when there is a significant risk or repeated intentional exposure of an infected instrument piercing the skin or making contact with mucous membranes. In the cosmetology field, broad-spectrum, hospital-grade and tuberculocidal disinfection is appropriate. For estheticians, however, sterilization is certainly a viable option because estheticians have intentional, repeated exposure to mucous membranes with facial needles and the like.

Methods of Sterilization

There are two primary methods of physical sterilization: (1) the steam autoclave, and (2) the dry heat cabinet. The steam autoclave, the most popular and the most preferred because of its proven history of sterilizing, is like a pressure cooker. When steam is injected into a chamber at high pressure, it is possible to raise the temperature above boiling water. If something is left in the autoclave long enough, the high pressure and high heat will penetrate into all of the nooks and crannies of the sterilized object, cooking all the microorganisms including the bacterial spore (the most resistant microbiological life form), and will kill eventually all living organisms.

Another physical method of sterilization is the use of dry heat, a method more like an oven than a pressure cooker. Objects are placed into an oven-like chamber and baked until all forms of life are dead.

There are several types of dry heat sterilizers sold and you should be very cautious when choosing and using them. The opinion of most authorities in the field of microbiology and disinfection insist rigorous precleaning is absolutely necessary before using the dry heat method, especially true when using the glass bead method. Should you fail to preclean all microscopic, organic matter off the instrument prior to using the dry heat method, the risk of contaminating the glass bead or dry heat chamber is extremely high. Even if the objects are sterilized after treatment, should you have failed to preclean thoroughly, then the instruments could become recontaminated when removing the instruments and actually recontaminated the sterile implement. To date, there is no available method to clean the glass beads themselves. The other disadvantage to these types of units is the lack of standardization of dwell time available for users of these types of machines. In other words, it takes some time for the unit to reach the proper operating temperature, and since instruments vary in size, thickness, and the like, there is neither an accurate sterilization time recommendation for each particular instrument nor is sterilization guaranteed. Additionally, when using a glass bead method, a portion of the instrument sticks out from the glass beads and this part of the object does not get sterilized.

When using any of these heat methods, one must be certain the objects to be sterilized can withstand the intense heat. Many plastic items, such as combs and brushes, will either melt or become deformed during the sterilization process. This is acceptable if you are rendering an object harmless prior to throwing it away, but is certainly not practical for reusable tools.

Chemical sterilization is another from of disinfection, a form much different from the physical methods. These chemicals may be administered as either liquids (glutaraldehyde or formaldehyde) or as a gas (ethylene oxide).

Ethylene oxide is a gas used in a pressurized chamber. Ethylene oxide gas is very hazardous to the environment and people. It is not recommend for use in the beauty industry. Only hospitals and laboratories have the ability to work with this highly toxic compound.

Glutaraldehyde and formaldehyde are liquid chemicals that can sterilize objects, but both take a long time to sterilize. Generally speaking, these methods usually take somewhere between six to ten hours to achieve sterilization. There are many problems with using these chemicals and they should be treated with utmost care. Never use them in a poorly ventilated room. These chemicals give off extremely hazardous, noxious gases that are irritating to the eyes, nose, lungs, throat, and mouth. As little as 0.2 parts per million of glutaraldehyde in the air will cause respiratory irritation. Additionally, the federal government has established a limit to the exposure of formaldehyde at 1.5 parts per million and an eight-hour period is the maximum acceptable exposure limit for this chemical.

If you must use glutaraldehyde to sterilize, always keep the lid on the container. Never leave the solution exposed to the air since the vapors can be harmful. Glutaraldehyde has an activator that is mixed into the chemical to make it active. The solution should be tested with a glutaraldehyde monitor kit (either a test kit or dip stick) once the solution is activated to ensure that there is at least 1.5 percent active glutaraldehyde left in solution. Should this percentage drop below 1.5 percent, discard the solution as it may not be working properly. Every glutaraldehyde has a shelf-life once it is activated. Most of these products are 14 or 28–30 day use products. Do not try to exceed these use times as the chemical may not work beyond the time period specified on the label.

Limits to Sterilization

As with every process, there are limitations to sterilization. For example, one cannot sterilize a room. Likewise, it would be difficult to sterilize a chair or table since large objects are difficult to sterilize. In order to truly sterilize something, first one must preclean the object thoroughly, and then remove any residue left behind by the cleaning process. Secondly, one must figure out how to handle the sterilized object once it has been removed from the chamber or bath without recontaminating it. This might include rinsing with sterile, distilled water, as is the case when using glutaraldehyde, because if you use tap water the sterilized object would then no longer be sterile. Time is also a limitation to using sterilization. Disinfection takes a few short minutes; whereas sterilization can take several hours.

Sterilizing and the Salon

Sterilizing does have its place in the salon. If the salon provides electrolysis or other treatments, repeatedly piercing the skin, then these implements and tools should be sterilized whenever possible. However, for routine use in the salon, sterilization is an expensive, risky method. Disinfection's broad-spectrum, hospital-grade, and tuberculocidal benefits are certainly the more practical choices. (Figure 6–1.)

FIGURE 6–1
The autoclave.

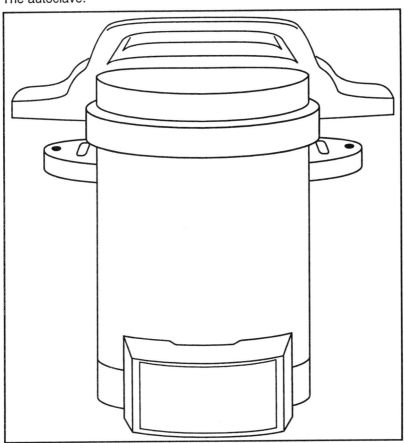

❏ REVIEW QUESTIONS

1. What are the two primary methods of physical sterilization?

2. How does the autoclave work to kill organisms?

3. Why is it necessary to preclean instruments before putting them in a dry heat cabinet?

4. What are some disadvantages of using glutaraldehyde and formaldehyde to sterilize objects?

5. How should sterilization be used in the salon?

SEVEN

AIDS, Hepatitis, and Personal Protection

❏ LEARNING OBJECTIVES

After completing this chapter, you should be able to:

■ Define AIDS.

■ Discuss the risks involved in the work place regarding the AIDS virus.

■ Define hepatitis.

■ Explain how to protect yourself and your clients from exposure to AIDS and hepatitis.

Introduction

Our work setting was much different years ago before we knew about acquired immune deficiency syndrome (AIDS) and before there were real concerns about hepatitis. In earlier times, we were much more concerned with measles, polio, and whooping cough, because these diseases could cause death to those infected with them. We have learned how to overcome these diseases; however, now society must contend with AIDS and hepatitis. In this chapter, we will learn about these diseases, how they are spread, and how to protect yourself from being exposed to them in your work place.

Questions and Answers Regarding AIDS

What is AIDS?

AIDS is a fatal disease caused by the human immunodeficiency virus (HIV). HIV invades and destroys specific cells in the body that normally fight off illness. This process of destroying the body's defenses can take several years. Individuals infected with HIV can live several years without showing any signs or symptoms of the disease. The most recent data seems to indicate HIV hides and multiplies in the lymph nodes for several years. HIV does not kill the victim. By destroying the body's defenses the infected person becomes prey to common microbes that other people's defenses can fight. The result is people infected with HIV die from diseases they caught and their bodies could not fight off.

At present, there is no cure for this disease. The amount of people becoming infected with HIV is growing rapidly, and scientists are working hard to find a cure.

Am I at risk if my client has AIDS?

This is a very difficult question to answer. However, the answer is generally no. If you are providing a service that does not puncture the skin, or come in contact with any blood or mucous membranes or exposed tissue, you are not at risk. A risk is created when there is direct exposure to blood, tissue, or other body fluids. If you are cutting the hair of a person who has the virus, and you accidently cut him and then cut yourself, and his blood gets into your cut, then it is possible you have been exposed and infected.

Accidental nicks, cuts, punctures, and scrapes do occur and one should take the necessary steps to keep them from occurring. If they do occur, then follow the instructions given later in this chapter.

If using a whirlpool bath, always be sure to decontaminate thoroughly between clients. Similarly, always decontaminate instruments and surfaces. Always wear gloves when decontaminating and never share your gloves with others.

How can I tell if my clients are carrying HIV?

Simply put, you cannot. This is why the approach called **universal precautions** has been adopted in the health-care field. The term and practice of universal precautions means you are to treat everyone as if they are infected since it is impossible to tell by merely looking at someone if they are infected. So, universal precautions means "playing it safe" by treating everyone the same (potentially infected). This healthcare field practice works for the beauty care industry as well.

By assuming your clients may have some form of infectious disease, it will assure you not to take any chances of becoming exposed to these diseases. It is just common sense telling you to be careful when doing your job so you do not become exposed.

What is hepatitis?

Hepatitis is an inflammatory disease of the liver. The liver is a vital organ within our body. Without it, we would die. The liver is responsible for a great number of functions including the manufacturing of chemicals helping us metabolize foods, drugs, and many of the chemicals the body produces. Probably the most easily seen symptom is jaundice. Jaundice is the yellowing of the skin and the whites of the eyes. It may take anywhere from three weeks to five months before jaundice and other symptoms appear.

Some forms of hepatitis are caused by viruses. Hepatitis A is a virus that can be transmitted through digestive secretions. Transmission has been traced back to contaminated food and utensils. It is possible to spread this virus through contaminated implements that have been in contact with saliva and other body fluids. This form of hepatitis is known as infectious hepatitis.

Another type of hepatitis is *hepatitis B*, which can be transmitted through contact with blood, blood serum, saliva, or other body fluids. This form of the disease is called serum Hepatitis and is far more serious than hepatitis A because of the greater incidence of more complications. However, both hepatitis A and hepatitis B should not be taken lightly.

All healthcare workers are now offered a hepatitis B vaccine routinely to prevent them form getting the virus. It would be very wise for all beauty care workers to obtain the vaccine for protection against the hepatitis B virus.

How can I protect myself from exposure to AIDS and hepatitis?

Protection from these viruses is merely common sense. As a basic rule, avoid touching any scrapes, nicks, or cuts your client may have. If a client looks jaundiced, ask her how she feels and if she has been evaluated for hepatitis. Should you cut or nick the skin, never blot up the blood with your bare hand. Put on a pair of disposable gloves before you touch the area. The same gloves colorists wear should give you adequate protection from exposure. Immediately after removing the gloves, wash and scrub your hands with an antimicrobial hand wash. Place all contaminated tools and instruments into a germicidal cleaner labeled effective against tuberculosis and follow all label directions. Decontaminate the counter where you were working and discard all towels, cotton, and other contaminated objects into a clean plastic bag. Tie it shut and place it into another plastic bag. Tie that shut and discard it into the trash outside of the salon.

Remember to always clean and disinfect after each client leaves.

❏ REVIEW QUESTIONS

1. What is AIDS?
2. How might one be exposed to AIDS while performing a salon service?
3. What is the theory of universal precautions?
4. What is hepatitis?
5. How is hepatitis A transmitted?
6. How is hepatitis B transmitted?
7. What precautions should one take to avoid exposure to AIDS and hepatitis in the salon?

C H A P T E R
E I G H T

Regulatory and Legal Requirements of Cleaning/Disinfection

□ LEARNING OBJECTIVES

After completing this chapter, you should be able to:

■ Identify the local and state agencies responsible for assuring that the consumer is not exposed to unsafe conditions.

■ Discuss the role of the United States Environmental Protection Agency in product registration.

■ Understand the importance of OSHA and the material safety data sheets.

■ Discuss the regulations of cleaning agents.

Introduction

There are several local, state, and federal agencies that regulate salons and beauty care establishments. These agencies direct how salons are to clean and disinfect their work places. Each of these agencies sets forth minimum cleanliness requirements for the salon and beauty care work place. There is some overlapping of responsibilities between these regulatory agencies, but the main objective of these agencies and laws is to protect both the employee and the public. Without this protection, there could be an increased risk of cross-infection and dangerous working conditions.

Regulatory Responsibilities

Local

In communities throughout the United States, there are several local agencies responsible for overseeing that the client is not exposed to unsafe conditions. Part of the responsibility is to make sure the places frequented by clients are free from the spread of germs. Your city or county health department is the agency responsible for setting minimum standards. If the health department suspects unsafe health conditions exist in a business, they can enter the business and inspect the premises. If there is evidence germs are being spread due to and caused by unsafe practices and conditions such as not disinfecting combs, brushes, nippers, shears, or any other piece of equipment in the salon, they can order the salon owner to correct the problem, or they may even temporarily close the salon until the deficiencies are corrected. Should this occur, there would probably be a fine and the possibility of negative publicity. This type of negative publicity would probably hurt the salon's business and cause clients to seek another salon.

Other local agencies which have responsibility in the beauty care industry are the business license bureau which can issue or revoke a license. Additionally there may be other local agencies in your area which monitor employee safety and health.

State Agencies

The most important state agencies of which you should be aware are the State Board of Cosmetology and Licensing, the State Board of Public Health, and any state occupational health and safety agencies that may be present within your state. State Boards of Cosmetology and Licensing are responsible for setting the minimum standards for proficiency of the employees working in the field. They are also responsible for establishing the minimum requirements for proper salon operation, including disinfection and sterilization. Many of the state boards seek the help of the State Board of Public Health and together they establish effective regulations.

The State Departments of Public Health provide guidelines for the cleaning disinfection of publicly frequented facilities including retail establishments. This agency can set the minimum requirements and standards for salons or they can provide guidance to State Boards of Cosmetology and Licensing. In either instance, this agency can help you to learn how to protect yourself as well as your clients.

Disinfectants, sterilants, and sanitizing agents are registered with each individual state. Each state sets the minimal standards of performance for these products and then registers these products for sale in the respective state. Most of the states follow federal regulations and registrations since they are more stringent and more comprehensive than most of the states. The State Department of Agriculture or the State Environmental Protection Agency are the registering agencies. This varies in each state.

If your state has an active Occupational Health and Safety Agency (OSHA)—or an agency with a similar name because this name can vary a bit—this agency has a great deal to do with protecting the employee from hazardous working conditions, such as being at risk from cross-infection. Many of these state agencies are now following the recently enacted guidelines published by OSHA (cf. "CPL 2–2.44C Bloodborne Pathogens Standard") for occupational exposure by healthcare workers for prevention of transmission of bloodborne pathogens (e.g., AIDS, hepatitis B, and other infectious agents). This includes accidental exposure as well. Many of these agencies are now adopting this plan for all workers in all occupations in which there is a potential for exposure to blood and or body fluids.

Federal Regulations and Requirements

The United States Environmental Protection Agency (EPA) is the federal agency responsible for registering all disinfecting agents, sterilants, and sanitizing agents. The EPA has set forth a complex set of requirements that manufacturers' products have to meet if they wish to obtain a product registration with the federal government. Their products must do what they say they will do on the product label and also must work under the conditions set forth on the product label in order to be granted this registration. When you look at any product that claims to kill germs on inanimate objects, always look for the EPA registration number. This number must be clearly displayed on the product label and may be abbreviated so that it looks like this: EPA Reg. No. 1043-62-062296. This number is your insurance policy that the product has met the minimal requirements specified on the product's label.

There are different levels for registering disinfectants/germicidal cleansers. Household products, those sold at the supermarket and other outlets, are the lowest level of disinfectant and don't really do a good job at all. They are formulated to be safe for use in the home and many of these products require using a lot of the concentrate to kill the germs present in tap water. When used in a salon, they become very expensive and are still not effective enough for salon needs.

The EPA's highest level of registration for disinfectants is the hospital grade category. This category or level requires the product to kill three kinds of organisms (*staphylococcus aureus, salmonella cholerasuis,* and *pseudomonas aeruginosa*) by following a strict set of laboratory-controlled conditions. The testing for these organisms can even be done in distilled water, which certainly does not replicate real-world conditions. (See chapter 5.) Should the manufacturer wish to add claims to the product label such as additional germ-killing ability as in tuberculosis, other bacteria, fungi, and viruses, more testing must be done to show that the product will, in fact, have microbial efficacy against these additional organisms. The EPA will then register these claims for inclusion on the product label as well. The same would be true when making efficacy claims for the HIV, and others.

The demonstration label shown in Figure 8–1 points out what you should look for when reading a disinfectant label. Note the claims and the test conditions shown.

Cleaning Agents: Who Regulates Them?

At the present time, cleaning agents are not regulated by any specific government agency. You are the judge of the products that you use. You are the only one who can determine if the products are working. Should you experience any problems while working with these products, contact the manufacturer of the particular product in question. Usually, they will try to help you. Should you have questions with regard to the safety of the particular cleaner, refer to the product material safety data sheet (MSDS)—also called OSHA Form No. 20. All manufacturers are required to supply these to you on all products containing potentially hazardous ingredients if you request them. Salons are required to have copies of MSDSs on every product containing potentially hazardous ingredients on file in the salon and available to all salon employees for their study. If you purchase your products from a professional supplier of products, they should be able to supply you with these sheets for your use.

There are many different agencies that either influence or regulate materials used to decontaminate salons. These agencies set the minimum requirements, not the ideal requirements that can and will protect you and your clients. You are the ultimate decision maker as to what will be used. You should always use the best products available. You are at risk even more than the client since you are exposed for hours each week; whereas the client is only there a short while. Remember, your health is at risk as well as your reputation so protect yourself the best you can.

FIGURE 8–1

A disinfectant label containing all the information regarding ingredients, directions for use, safety precautions, storage, and disposal.

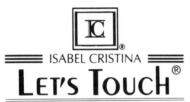

=== ISABEL CRISTINA ===

LET'S TOUCH®

HOSPITAL GRADE, INSTRUMENT
DISINFECTANT FOR DISINFECTION AND STORAGE OF
INSTRUMENTS

BACTERIOCIDAL • FUNGICIDAL • STAPHYLOCIDAL
PSEUDOMONICIDAL • VIRUCIDAL • TUBERCULOCIDAL

EPA Reg. No. 1043-36-062296
EPA Est. No. 11563-MI-1

Active Ingredients:

o-Benzyl-p-chlorophenol 5.25%
o-Phenyphenol 1.00%
INERT INGREDIENTS 93.75%

MINIMUM USE - DILUTION CONFIRMATION
(A.O.A.C. - 10 Min. - 20C)
S. choleraesuis - 1:32, S. aureus - 1:32,
Ps. aeruginosa - 1:32

A 1:32 Dilution is effective against M. Tuberculosis on hard, inanimate surfaces in 10 minutes at 20 C. Remove heavy soil or gross filth and thoroughly clean surfaces.

LET'S TOUCH is an E.P.A. Registered, Hospital Grade, Instrument Disinfectant. This product is TO BE USED ONLY at a 1:32 Dilution with Water for cold disinfection of precleaned instruments. The 1:32 DILUTION KILLS pathogenic bacteria and fungi such as C. albicans (yeast), Trichophyton mentagrophytes (Athletes Foot), S. aureus, S. choleraesuis, Ps. aeruginosa, and Mycobacterium Tuberculosis (effective in 10 min. at 20 C). LET'S TOUCH is virucidal against Influenza A1 (NJ), Influenza A2 (Hong Kong), Type 2 Adenovirus, Vaccinia, and Herpes Simplex 1 & 2 on hard, innanimate surfaces in 10 minutes at 20 C.

CAUTION: KEEP OUT OF REACH OF CHILDREN

STATEMENT OF PRACTICAL TREATMENT
Incase of eye contact, flush with water for 15 minutes. Get prompt medical attention. For skin contact, flush with water. See back panel for additional precautionary statements and directions for use.
CONTENTS: 1 FL. OZ. (29.5 ML)

PRECAUTIONARY STATEMENTS
HAZARD TO HUMANS AND DOMESTIC ANIMALS
CAUTION: Harmful if swallowed. Avoid prolonged skin contact and avoid splashing in eyes. Wash eyes with large amounts of flowing water if exposed.

DIRECTIONS FOR USE -

It is a violation of Federal law to use this product in a manner inconsistent with its labeling.

1. Thoroughly clean and rinse instruments and or containers prior to first use of this product to remove any excess organic residue present, then rough dry.
2. Fill container with 1 quart (32 oz.) of tap water.
3. Grasp packet at upper corner at the notch.
4. Tear packet open along the top in the direction of the notch.
5. Pour contents into premeasured water and mix. Take precautions so as to avoid any direct contact with the undiluted disinfectant. The removal of heavy soils (hair, oils and residues) and the cleaning of all surfaces prior to application of this product is required.

INSTRUMENT DISINFECTION -
1. After cleaning, immerse articles and wet all surfaces thoroughly in a 1:32 solution for 10 Minutes.
2. Rinse and Dry.
To remove residue of previous disinfectant thoroughly clean and rinse instruments prior to first use of this product.
Prepare a new solution daily or when solution turns cloudy or dirty for disinfecting precleaned items.

METAL INSTRUMENT STORAGE -
A 1:32 solution is noncorrosive and does not rust, dull, or otherwise stain or attack quality metal instruments. This solution is not for prolonged storage of plastic or rubber items. 10 minute disinfection of plastic or rubber items is acceptable. This is a complete product. Do not add any other chemicals to it. Use only as directed. If frozen, thaw and remix before use.

STORAGE AND DISPOSAL
PROHIBITIONS: Open dumping is prohibited. Do not contaminate water, food or feed by storage or disposal. Pesticide Disposal: This germicide, its solutions or rinsings from empty containers, should be disposed of in a toilet or service sink served by a sanitary sewer.
CONTAINER DISPOSAL: Do not reuse empty pouch. Wrap pouch and put in trash.   6401-12A

 === ISABEL CRISTINA ===
"Beauty Care Products For The Educated Professional"
POB 3599 TEANECK, NJ 07666
800-247-4130   201-489-1700
(Outside NJ)   (In NJ)

FRONT   **BACK**

❏ REVIEW QUESTIONS

1. Name the most important state agencies that are responsible for overseeing that the consumer is not exposed to unsafe conditions.

2. What are the roles of the State Boards of Cosmetology and Licensing and the State departments of Public Health with regard to the salon environment?

3. How does OSHA protect employees from hazardous working conditions?

4. How can one determine if a product will kill germs on inanimate objects?

5. How does one obtain copies of material safety data sheets (MSDS)?

6. When are salons required to have material safety data sheets on hand?

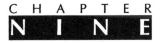

Protocol
for
Salons

❏ LEARNING OBJECTIVES

After completing this chapter, you should be able to:

■ Describe the acceptable visual appearance of salon professionals.

■ Discuss the elements that make up a safe, healthy, and professional salon environment.

■ Describe the proper use and disinfection of salon implements, tools, and equipment.

■ Use the salon protection checklist for clients and operators.

Introduction

Since we are a service-oriented profession, we must keep in mind four very important facts:

1. Our visual appearance, work performance, and salon environment communicate many things about us to the clients

2. Clients watch everything we do, hear everything we say, and repeat stories about us to other people

3. We want to keep our clients satisfied so they will return to us over and over

4. We must use the highest standards of care possible to protect ourselves and our clients from the chances of cross-contamination of infectious diseases.

The Salon Environment

Clients should expect to see operators with a neat and clean appearance. The salon should be temperature-controlled, well lighted, and comfortably heated or air conditioned. The salon should also be ventilated and purified for any potential contagens and odors.

The salon should have properly disinfected floors and windows, salon furniture, counters and stations, restrooms (supplied with liquid soap pump dispensers and individual paper towels), sinks, and the like. The walls, curtains, and floor coverings in a salon must be washed and cleaned regularly. The premises must be kept free from rodents, vermin, flies, and insects. There should be no hair, cotton, or other waste materials on the floor.

Towels and linens should always be clean and stored in a closed cabinet. Soiled towels and linens should be in a closed container, away from clean towels and linens.

There should be clean manicure bowls, foot baths, skin care equipment, and tanning beds. Instrument jars should be clean and instruments should be fully immersed in a clean, hospital-grade, tuberculocidal disinfectant solution. Combs, brushes, nail files, nippers, and shears should also be properly disinfected in an EPA-registered, broad-spectrum, hospital-grade, tuberculocidal disinfectant.

Any lotions, ointments, and creams should be kept in closed containers and re-covered after use.

All disposable items should be thrown away in sealed plastic bags.

Food should be stored and eaten in a separate area from service stations.

Animals should not be on the premises.

Operators should wear clean clothes at all times. Operators should wash their hands thoroughly, before and after each client, and after using the bathroom or eating. Preferably you should use an antimicrobial handsoap listed with FDA and with an NDC number on the label (e.g., NDC 00176209814). A clean, disinfected towel should be used for each client, or use disposable paper towels. Towels and linens should be replaced between clients and stored in a closed cabinet. Soiled towels and linens must be placed immediately in closed containers. Headrest coverings and neck strips must be changed for each client. The shampoo cape should not come in contact with the client's skin.

Implements, Tools, and Equipment

All implements should be disinfected after each use. If a one-step germicidal cleaner is not used, all implements should be washed in hot, soapy water. (All instruments, including files, nippers, and shears should be scrubbed to clear them of particles of nail, skin, hair, and creams.) They should be rinsed thoroughly with clean water, and placed into a disinfection solution of an EPA-registered, broad-spectrum, hospital-grade, tuberculocidal type. If the solution does not allow for storage of instruments in it at all times, they should then be rinsed, dried and placed in a dustproof, germ-free area until the next use, such as an Ultraviolet light cabinet. To ensure germicidal activity (germ killing), frequently change the solution in the wet disinfectant (whenever cloudy or dirty).

Soiled combs, brushes, towels, or other used material must be removed from the tops of work stations immediately after use. Combs or implements must not be carried in pockets of the uniform. Clippies, hairpins, bobby pins, or curlers must not be placed in the mouth; these items must be disinfected after each use. Objects dropped on the floor are not to be used until they are cleaned and disinfected.

Lotions, ointments, and creams must be kept in clean, closed containers. Clients should not be allowed to dip into these with their hands. A cream spatula must be used for each dipping. Use a new spatula, each time, to remove cosmetics from the jars. Use disposable cotton pads to apply lotions and powders. Re-cover all containers after each use. Discard emery boards after use on a client if you cannot disinfect the board or if the board comes into contact with blood, pus, or an infected nail.

All environmental surfaces in the salon should be disinfected with an EPA-registered, broad-spectrum, hospital-grade, tuberculocidal disinfectant, including counters and stations, restrooms and sinks, floors and windows, skin care equipment, and tanning beds. Always follow the manufacturer's label directions for correct application and preparation instructions.

All disposable items should be thrown out between clients and placed in a sealed plastic bag, at the end of each day.

Important Reminders

- All operators should maintain a neat, clean appearance.

- Salon should be temperature-controlled, well lighted, comfortably heated/air-conditioned, ventilated and air-purified for potential contagens and offensive odors.

- All salons must have hot and cold running water. Drinking facilities should be provided with individual, disposable paper cups or a water fountain.

- The premises must be kept free from rodents, vermin, flies, and insects.

- The salon must have properly disinfected floors, windows, salon furniture, counters, stations, restrooms (supplied with liquid soap pump dispensers and individual paper towels), and sinks.

■ The walls, curtains, and floor coverings in a salon must be kept clean.

■ All towels and linens must be clean.

■ Clean manicure bowls, foot baths, skin care equipment, tanning beds, and the like.

■ Be sure to clean and disinfect instrument jars and all instruments and then fully immerse them in an EPA-registered, broad-spectrum, hospital-grade, tuberculocidal solution. Follow the specific label instructions exactly.

■ Properly disinfect all combs, brushes, nail files, nippers, shears, and all other instruments in an EPA-registered, broad-spectrum, hospital-grade, tuberculocidal solution.

■ Keep all lotions, ointments, and creams in closed containers.

■ Remove all hair, cotton, and other waste materials from the floor immediately and deposit the waste into closed containers. Waste bags should be removed frequently from the premises in sealed plastic bags and discarded properly.

■ All foods and drinks should be consumed in a place separate from the work station areas.

■ No animals should be allowed on the premises.

■ Operators should wear clean clothes at all times.

■ Operators should always wear gloves.

■ Operators must wash their hands thoroughly with an antimicrobial handwash before and after each client, and after using the bathroom and eating.

■ Between clients, be sure to replace and have clean, disinfected towels and linens.

■ Instruments should be washed in hot, soapy water, then rinsed thoroughly, and immersed in a solution that is EPA-registered, broad-spectrum, hospital-grade, and tuberculocidal.

- Files, nippers, shears, and all other instruments must be scrubbed to remove all particles of nail, skin, hair, creams, and the like. Then the instruments must be rinsed and immersed in a disinfection solution that is EPA-registered, broad-spectrum, hospital-grade, and tuberculocidal.

- It is highly preferred to store all disinfected instruments in an EPA-registered, broad-spectrum, hospital-grade, and tuberculocidal disinfectant solution; if this is not possible, then the instruments should placed in a germ-free area until their next use.

- All soiled combs, brushes, towels, and other materials must be removed from the tops of all work stations immediately after their use.

- No combs or implements are to be carried in any pockets.

- Do not place clippies, hairpins, curlers, or bobby pins in your mouth.

- All clippies, hairpins, curlers, and bobby pins must be disinfected after each use.

- All objects dropped on the floor are not to be used until they are disinfected in an EPA-registered, broad-spectrum, hospital-grade, and tuberculocidal disinfectant.

- All chemical solutions in wet disinfection baths should be changed frequently, when either cloudy or dirty, to assure germicidal activity (germ-killing ability).

- Manicure bowls, foot baths, skin care equipment, tanning beds, and the like should be disinfected between clients.

- Lotions, ointments, and creams must be kept in clean, closed containers and properly labeled.

- Clients should not be allowed to dip either their hands or feet into lotions, ointments, or creams. Cream spatulas must be used for each dipping. Use a new spatula each time you remove cosmetics from jars. Disposable cotton pads should be used to apply lotions and powders. Re-cover cosmetic containers after each use. Discard emery boards after use on a client if they cannot be disinfected.

■ All environmental surfaces, including counters and stations, restrooms, and sinks, floors and windows, skin care equipment, and tanning beds should be disinfected with an EPA-registered, broad-spectrum, hospital-grade tuberculocidal disinfectant.

■ All disposable items should be thrown out between clients, placed in sealed plastic bags and discarded daily.

■ Each client must receive new, clean headrest coverings and neck strips.

■ Operators should not be working or at the salon with colds, viruses, flu, or any other contagious illness.

■ Any cuts, wounds, blisters, open sores, and the like should be bandaged and kept from coming into contact with clients.

❏ REVIEW QUESTIONS

1. What rule should be observed regarding the appearance of salon professionals?

2. Describe the ideal environmental air quality of the salon.

3. How should combs, brushes, nail files and other instruments be disinfected?

4. What should be observed regarding food in the salon?

5. What is the preferred hand soap to use in the salon?

6. How should lotions, ointments, creams, and the like be used and stored?

7. How should disinfected instruments be stored?

8. What is the best way to discard disposable items?

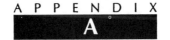
Product Consideration Factors

Safety

EPA-Registered

Labeled Use Instructions

Caution Statements

Ultra Convenience Package

Accurate Dispenser Provided

Closed System

Toxicity Data Available

Uses

Used on Food Contact Surfaces

Used in Automatic Scrubbers

Used in Mechanical Application Devices

Used on Surgical and Medical Equipment

UL Approved For Use on Conductive Floors

Effectiveness

EPA-Registered

AOAC Test Data

Detergent Sanitizer Tested

AOAC Available Chlorine Equivalency Test

Public Health Accepted

Hard Water Effective by Use-Dilution Test

Organic Matter Activity Test Data

Detergency (Gardner Washability Test)

5% Serum Effective by Use-Dilution Test

BROAD SPRECTRUM GERMICIDE (See Technical Data)

    AOAC Use-Dilution Test Data

    Pseudomonas aeruginosa

    Salmonella choleraesuis

    Staphylococcus aureus

    Other Pathogenic Organisms

Tuberculocidal

Fungicidal

Virucidal

Economy

One-Step Germicidal Cleaner

Freight-Storage-Handling Savings

Accurate Dispensing

Use Solution = Gallon Cost ÷ Dilution Factor

Service

Program Implementation

In-Service Training

Training Aids and Tools

Program Follow Up

Technical Consultations

Research and Development

Quality Controls

Manufacturer's Reputation

National Representation

Product Availability

B

Advantages and Disadvantages of Biocidal Agents

Phenolic Compounds

Advantages

1. Generally fungicidal
2. Generally tuberculocidal
3. Broad-spectrum biocidal activity
4. Visually stable and very soluble
5. Can be effective in the presence of organic matter
6. Established use history
7. Hard water effective
8. Newer formulae safe on food contact surfaces
9. Temporary "bonds"
10. Can be bacteriostatic

Disadvantages

1. Effectiveness can be reduced by the presence of alkaline pH, natural soap, or some organic materials
2. Some areas have disposal restrictions against phenolics
3. Medicinal odor
4. Not sporicidal
5. Cannot be combined with cationic wetting agents
6. Can swell natural rubber and some plastics

Quaternary Ammonium Chloride Compounds (Quats)

Advantages

1. Exceptionally good against gram positive
2. Bacteriostatic in high concentrations
3. Usually stable and very soluble
4. Very compatible with detergents (cationic wetting agents)
5. Good deodorizers
6. May be used on food preparation surfaces
7. Non-staining

Disadvantages

1. Not generally tuberculocidal
2. Not sporicidal
3. Not effective against some viruses
4. Can be affected by hard water
5. Can be affected by organic loads
6. Permanent "bonds" on metal (discoloration)

Iodophors

Advantages

1. Affected by hard water
2. Very effective against some viruses
3. Some may be used on food preparation surfaces
4. Quick microbial kill
5. Excellent against gram positive and some gram negative bacteria

Disadvantages

1. Not good cleaners
2. May stain
3. May be irritating to mucous membranes
4. Inactivated by exposure to ultraviolet light or heat
5. Inactivated by organic material
6. Water sensitive

Chlorine Compounds

Advantages

1. Relatively quick microbial kill
2. Can be tuberculocidal
3. May be used on food preparation surfaces

Disadvantages

1. Effectiveness is pH dependent
2. Inactivated in heavy organic material, exposure to ultraviolet light or heat
3. Objectionable taste and odor unless strictly controlled
4. Not sporicidal
5. Corrosive to metals
6. Not good cleaners

Glutaraldehyde

Advantages

1. Non-staining, relatively non-corrosive
2. Sporicidal, tuberculocidal, virucidal
3. Usable as a sterilizer on plastics, rubber, lenses, stainless steel, and other items that cannot be autoclaved.
4. Some formulas can be reused for 14–28 days.

Disadvantages

1. Not extremely stable in solution
2. Usually has to be in alkaline solution
3. Can be irritating to sensitive skin
4. Inactivated by heavy organic matter
5. May be irritating to mucous membranes
6. Inhalation toxicity starts at 0.5 p.p.m.

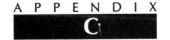

APPENDIX
C

Characteristics of Particles and Particle Dispersoids

Reprinted with permission from C.E. Lapple, SRI Journal, 5, 94 (Third Quarter, 1961).

Particle Diameter, microns (μ)

Equivalent Sizes		

(1mμ) 0.001 · (1μ) · 0.1 · 1 · 10 · 100 · (1mm) 1,000 · (1cm) 10,000

Angström Units, Å — 10 · 100 · 1,000 · 10,000

Theoretical Mesh (Used very infrequently): 625 · 1,250 · 2,500 · 5,000 · 10,000

Tyler Screen Mesh · U.S. Screen Mesh

Electromagnetic Waves: X-Rays — Ultraviolet — Visible — Near Infrared — Solar Radiation — Far Infrared — Microwaves (Radar, etc.)

Technical Definitions:
- Gas Dispersoids — Solid: Fume — Dust
- Liquid: Mist — Spray
- Soil: Clay · Silt · Fine Sand · Coarse Sand · Gravel (Atterberg or International Std. Classification System adopted by Internat. Soc. Soil Sci. Since 1934)

Common Atmospheric Dispersoids: Smog · Clouds and Fog · Mist · Drizzle · Rain

Typical Particles and Gas Dispersoids:
Rosin Smoke · Oil Smokes · Tobacco Smoke · Metallurgical Dusts and Fumes · Ammonium Chloride Fume · Sulfuric Concentrator Mist · Contact Sulfuric Mist · Alkali Fume · Spray Dried Milk · Ground Talc · Plant Spores · Pollens · Milled Flour · Fertilizer, Ground Limestone · Fly Ash · Coal Dust · Cement Dust · Pulverized Coal · Flotation Ores · Beach Sand · Hydraulic Nozzle Drops · Carbon Black · Paint Pigments · Zinc Oxide Fume · Colloidal Silica · Insecticide Dusts · Atmospheric Dust · Sea Salt Nuclei · Nebulizer Drops · Lung Damaging Dust · Pneumatic Nozzle Drops · Human Hair · Aitken Nuclei · Combustion Nuclei · Red Blood Cell Diameter (Adults): 7.5μ ± 0.3μ · Bacteria · Viruses

Gas Molecules*: C₄H₁₀ · C₂H₆ · SO₂ · Cl₂ · CO₂ · HCl · F₂ · CH₄ · O₂ · H₂O · N₂ · H₂ · CO

*Molecular diameters calculated from viscosity data at 0°C.

Particle Diameter, microns (μ)

0.0001	0.001 (1mμ)	0.01	0.1	1
				10	100	1,000 (1mm.)	10,000 (1cm.)

Methods for Particle Size Analysis
— Impingers —
— Ultramicroscope + —
— Electron Microscope —
— X-Ray Diffraction + —
— Adsorption + —
— Nuclei Counter —
— Ultracentrifuge —
— Centrifuge —
— Turbidimetry ++ —
— Sedimentation —
— Elutriation —
— Microscope + —
— Electroformed Sieves —
— Sieving —
— Permeability + —
— Light Scattering ++ —
— Scanners —
— Electrical Conductivity —
— Visible to Eye —
— Machine Tools (Micrometers, Calipers, etc.) —

+ Furnishes average particle diameter but no size distribution.
++ Size distribution may be obtained by special calibration.

Types of Gas Cleaning Equipment
— Ultrasonics (very limited industrial application) —
— Settling Chambers —
— Centrifugal Separators —
— Liquid Scrubbers —
— Cloth Collectors —
— Packed Beds —
— Common Air Filters —
— Impingement Separators —
— Mechanical Separators —
— High Efficiency Air Filters —
— Thermal Precipitation (used only for sampling) —
— Electrical Precipitators —

Terminal Gravitational Settling* [for spheres, sp. gr. 2.0]	Reynolds Number	In Air at 25°C. 1 atm.
	Settling Velocity, cm/sec.	
	Reynolds Number	In Water at 25°C.
	Settling Velocity, cm/sec.	

| **Particle Diffusion Coefficient,*** cm²/sec. | In Air at 25°C. 1 atm. |
| | In Water at 25°C. |

*Stokes-Cunningham factor included in values given for air but not included for water

PREPARED BY C.E. LAPPLE

Answers to Review Questions

Chapter 1   A Historical Look at Germs

1. Approximately one third of the population died from *Yursinia pestis*, the microorganism (bacteria) responsible for the disease.

2. The fundamental rule is to clean and disinfect to protect all.

3. The individual staff member is responsible for keeping the work environment clean and safe from soils and germs.

4. Bar soap will support the growth of microorganisms. That is why liquid hand soap dispensed from a pump is preferred.

5. The principles of cleaning and decontamination are the essential building blocks providing cosmetologists and clients the protection from the risk of cross-infection.

Chapter 2   The Microbial World

1. Microbiology is the branch of science studying the microbial world (living organisms—microbes or microorganisms—unseen by the naked eye).

2. Anthony van Leeuenhoek is the father of the microscope.

3. Pasteurization heats materials to a temperature destroying most of the microbes.

4. *Phenol* (a chemical from coal tar called carbolic acid) was used to wash surgical instruments, patients' skin, the operating table and the surgeons' hands. Also bandages and dressings soaked in *phenol* were used. The result was that many patients survived as a result of these precautions.

5. A round or marble-shaped bacterium is referred to as coccus. An example of the use of coccus is streptoccus, as in *strepococcus faecialis*, the organism responsible for causing strep throat. Rod-shaped bacteria are referred to as bacillus and the organism causing tuberculosis has this shape. Another bacterial shape is the spiral, known as spirochetes. One of these organisms is responsible for causing syphilis.

6. The gram staining technique helps make organisms visible under a microscope.

7. Bacteria have a distinct cell wall, a nucleus containing the genetic code, cytoplasmic constituents filling the cell (its guts), a possible way of moving around (a tail or a whip called a flagellum), and anchoring strands (fimbri) allowing the bacteria to hold on to an object.

8. Some fungal infections include nail fungus, ringworm, athlete's foot, jock itch.

9. Viral particles may be on a droplet of saliva when someone sneezes of coughs, or they may be deposited on an inanimate object like a countertop or scissors. They may be on a door handle to a shop or on the handle of clippers.

Chapter 3   Sources of Contamination and Disease

1. Pathogens are disease-producing organisms. Opportunistic microorganisms are microbes that do not necessarily cause illness; but if the circumstances prevail, and

a person does not have the ability to fight off the microbes, they can be infected.

2. The shampoo sink is notorious for contamination with many different kinds of microorganisms. The implements used during a client's salon visit, like scissors, files, nippers, and brushes, are other sources of contamination.

3. OSHA finds blood is a prime source of pathogens. OSHA has issued a legal requirement for protecting all healthcare workers, even those remotely exposed to blood.

4. Colds are caused by virus particles invading the tissues of the respiratory tract. Colds can be spread by either inhaling contaminated droplets in the air, called airborne transmission, or by touching a contaminated surface, and then touching your eyes, mouth, or a mucous membrane.

5. If an infected person with athlete's foot walks barefoot on a floor, the infected feet will leave contaminated particles (fungal spores) so the next barefoot person who walks on the same floor might be infected.

Chapter 4   Breaking the Chain of Cross-Infection

1. Infection control is a combination of basic knowledge of what causes infection, how to control or prevent infection from occurring, and common sense. Infection control requires a working understanding of the necessary requisites of the principles of sanitization and personal hygiene.

2. Cleaning is the removal of undesirable substances from a surface.

3. Emulsification is the process of lifting soils off the surface and suspending them so they may be rinsed off.

4. Tallow or vegetable oil is reacted with lye to produce natural soap. This process is called hydrolysis or saponification.

5. Soaps start out as some form of fat. The fat is reacted with lye and other materials are added to the mixture to make it feel better, be less aggressive, or smell good. Soaps leave residue. Detergents can break down the surface tension of water and soils, emulsifying and dissolving soils; but they cannot convert fatty soils into soap. Detergents are generally free rinsing.

6. The four levels of disinfection efficacy are: 1. limited disinfection (very low level); 2. general disinfection (low level); 3. hospital-grade disinfection (plain); and 4. hospital-gradetuberculocidal disinfection (ideal).

7. Hospital-level tuberculocidal is the ideal level of disinfection available. It is a broad spectrum disinfection suitable for the salon infection control. It kills TB which has a very hard outer coat which is more difficult to penetrate than Pseudomonas.

8. Sterilization kills all forms of biologic life, including the bacterial spore; whereas disinfection does not.

9. Sterilization is generally accomplished by using a sterilizing chamber, such as a steam autoclave, which rises the temperature and pressure so high that all life is destroyed. Other methods of sterilization include the use of ethylene oxide gas in a chamber, or extremely dangerous chemicals, which should be handled under a chemical fume hood by experts

10. A room cannot be sterilized. If you want to sterilize equipment, cleaning and disinfecting will render them safe to handle before sterilizing anyway. Sanitizing does not kill the organism completely and is wasteful of supplies and labor. Disinfection kills germs without creating a hostile environment in the salon.

11. Sanitizing requires you first wash the surface with a cleaner, rinse with water, and then apply an agent which does not kill 100 percent of the microbes.

Chapter 5   Decontaminating Materials and Procedures

1. One-step germicidal cleaners are formulated to clean, disinfect, and deodorize simultaneously. Two-step cleaners, like bleach, must be used in conjunction with other substances like water. Therefore, you must clean the surface with a cleaning agent, rinse, and apply bleach to the surface. Using two-step products like bleach is rather impractical because it is costly and labor intensive.

2. The active ingredients used to formulate commercially available one-step and two-step disinfection products include: phenols or phenolics, quaternary ammonium compounds (quats), alcohol, bleach or hypochlorite, iodine or iodophor based, pine oil based, and mild acids, such as vinegar.

3. The Environmental Protection Agency (EPA), is the governmental regulating agency responsible disinfectants, sterilants, and sanitizing agents.

4. Biocldal efficacy is one of the key points used by the EPA to classify the strength of disinfecting agents.

5. Biocidal efficacy is the ability to kill specific organisms.

6. Advantages of phenolic compounds include: they have an extremely broad range of germ-killing activity; they are not affected by organic matter as much as other compounds; and they have a proven history.

7. Advantages of quats include: they are excellent cleaning agents and are very compatible with many other wetting agents; they have excellent disinfecting properties against gram positive bacteria and are very effective on easy-to-kill bacteria; they are relatively non-toxic in solution; they may be used on food preparation surfaces; and they have excellent deodorizing properties.

8. Advantages of iodophor-based disinfectants include: they are very effective against some viruses and are excellent against the gram positive and some gram nega-

tive bacteria; some may be used to sanitize food contact surfaces; they may be used to disinfect drinking water; and they have very quick microbial killing times.

9. Alcohols are not sterilants and do not kill flu-like viruses.

10. The result could be disastrous or even bring death. A form of nerve gas is made by mixing bleach, vinegar, and TSP (the cleaning agent found in many household cleaners). When used by itself, TSP can do the job;, consequently, a mixture of bleach and TSP can kill people.

11. The sevens factors affecting how a disinfectant will work in the salon are: (1) dilution of the solution; (2) dwell time; (3) water; (4) types of soils; (5) pH; (6) temperature; and (7) the user.

12. Minerals in the water govern the hardness or softness of the water. Very hard water leaves a white ring or film on surfaces. Softened water makes cleaning skin, hair, and all inanimate objects easier, providing excellent results.

13. The ideal pH range for germicidal cleaning agents and/ or disinfectants is between 2.6 and 3.2 on the acid side of the pH scale and between 10 and 11 on the alkaline side of the pH scale.

Chapter 6   Sterilization

1. The two primary methods of physical sterilization are: (1) the steam autoclave, and (2) the dry heat cabinet.

2. High pressure and high heat penetrates into all the nooks and crannies of the sterilized object, cooking all the microorganisms including the bacterial spore (the most resistant microbiological life form), and eventually killing all living organisms.

3. Without precleaning all microscopic, organic matter from instruments prior to using the dry heat method, the risk of contaminating the glass bead or dry heat chamber is extremely high.

4. Glutaraldehyde and formaldehyde take a long time to sterilize. These chemicals also give off extremely hazardous, noxious gases, which are irritating to the eyes, nose, lungs, throat, and mouth.

5. If the salon provides services as electrolysis or other treatments, repeatedly piercing the skin, then these implements and tools should be sterilized whenever possible. However, for routine use in the salon, sterilization is an expensive, risky method.

Chapter 7   AIDS, Hepatitis, and Personal Protection

1. AIDS is a fatal disease caused by the human immunodeficiency virus (HIV). HIV invades and destroys specific cells in the body that would normally fight off illness.

2. 2. If you trim the hair of someone who has the virus, and you accidently cut him and then cut yourself, and their blood gets into your cut, then it is very possible you will be exposed and infected.

3. Universal precaution means you are to treat everyone as if they are infected, since it is impossible to tell by merely looking at someone if they are infected.

4. Hepatitis is an inflammatory disease of the liver.

5. Hepatitis A is a virus that can be transmitted through digestive secretions. Transmission may be traced back to contaminated food and utensils.

6. Hepatitis B can be transmitted through contact with blood, blood serum, saliva, or other body fluids.

7. Avoid touching any scrapes, nicks, or cuts a client may have. Wear disposable gloves whenever possible. Always clean and disinfect when a client leaves.

Chapter 8   Regulatory and Legal Requirements of Cleaning/Disinfection

1. The most important state agencies are the State Boards of Cosmetology and Licensing, the State Board of Public Health, and any state occupational health and safety agencies present in your particular state.

2. State Boards of Cosmetology and Licensing are responsible for setting the minimum standards for proficiency of the employees working in the field. They are also responsible for establishing the minimum requirements for proper salon operation, including disinfection and sterilization. The State Departments of Public Health provide guidelines for the cleaning and disinfection of publicly frequented facilities.

3. OSHA publishes guidelines for occupational exposure by healthcare workers for prevention of transmission of bloodborne pathogens. These guidelines can be adopted for all workers in occupations in which there is a potential for exposure to blood and/or body fluids.

4. When you look at any product that claims to kill germs on inanimate objects, always look for the EPA registration number displayed on the product.

5. All manufacturers are required to supply MSDSs on all products that contain potentially hazardous ingredients.

6. Salons are required to have copies of MSDSs on every product that contains potentially hazardous ingredients on file in the salon and available to all salon employees for their study.

Chapter 9   Protocol for Salons

1. All salon professionals should maintain a neat, clean appearance.

2. The salon should be temperature-controlled, well lighted, comfortably heated or air conditioned, ventilated and air-purified for potential contagens and offensive odors.

3. Combs, brushes, nail files, nippers, shears, and all other instruments should be disinfected in an EPA-registered, broad-spectrum, hospital-grade, tuberculocidal solution.

4. All foods and drinks should be consumed in a place separate from the work station areas.

5. An antimicrobial hand soap listed with the FDA and with an NDC number on the label should be used in the salon.

6. Lotions, ointments, and creams must be kept in clean, closed containers. Clients should not be allowed to dip into these with their hands. Cream spatulas must be used for each dipping. A new spatula must be used each time to remove cosmetics from jars. Disposable cotton pads should be used to apply lotions and powders.

7. Preferably, all disinfected instruments should be stored in an EPA-registered, broad-spectrum, hospital-grade, and tuberculocidal disinfectant solution. If this is not possible, then the instruments should be placed in a germ-free area until their next use.

8. All disposable items should be thrown out after used for a client, placed in in sealed plastic bags and discarded daily.

Glossary

Acids:
Materials with a pH value below 7.

Active ingredients:
the materials that kill germs.

Aerobe (ER ohb):
a microorganism that will grow in the presence of oxygen.

Aerobic bacteria:
bacteria living in oxygen-rich environments (such as air).

Aerosol:
a suspension of fine solid or liquid particles in air or gas, as a fog, smoke, or mist.

Agar:
a gelatinous material extracted from seaweed that is used to form the solid base for bacteriological culture medium.

Airborne transmission:
contracting a disease by inhaling contaminated droplets in the air.

Anaerobe:
a microorganism that can live without air.

Anaerobic bacteria:
bacteria needing no air.

Bacillus (pl., bacilli):
rod-shaped bacterium.

Bacterium (pl., bacteria):
one-celled microorganisms with no chlorophyll that multiply by simple division.

Beneficial microorganism:
used to make bread dough rise, ferment spirits, and breakdown organic matter.

Binary fission:
"the making of two by splitting in half"; the method by which bacteria reproduce.

Biocidal efficacy:
the ability to kill the organisms.

Broad-spectrum efficacy:
possessing a wide range of germ-killing activity.

Carriers:
people who carry and transmit disease germs, especially one who is immune to the germs carried.

Chlorophyll
the substance that makes plants green; the key component in photosynthesis.

Cleaning:
the removal of undesirable substances from a surface.

Cleaning agents:
chemicals that assist cleaning.

Coccus (pl., cocci):
a round or marble-shaped bacterium.

Coliform bacteria:
bacteria that ferment lactose sugar with the production of gas, do not produce spores, are gram negatively stained, and may either grow aerobically or anaerobically. (Escherichia coli is the most typical of this group.)

Colony:

the mass of bacterial cells observed on the surface of solid culture medium that may be large enough to be seen without magnification. Bacteria normally do not produce colonies on typical hospital environmental surfaces. A colony forms as the result of the growth of bacterial cells usually during an incubation period of from 24–48 hours at temperatures above 25°C. The "colony count" refers to the number of colonies observed after incubation on petri dishes or rodac plates that relates to the original number of bacterial cells deposited on the agar medium.

Communicable disease:

a disease or infection that may be transmitted from one person to another by various means.

Contagious:

a state whereby a disease or infection may be transmitted or spread from one person to another; also refers to a microorganism that is capable of causing a communicable disease.

Contamination:

the occurrence of microorganisms on surfaces or in air where their presence is undesirable for health or esthetic reasons. Not to be confused with infection or contagion.

Cross-infection:

the act of transmitting an infection from one infected person to another. Also refers to becoming infected by a microorganism picked up by contact with a surface (or air) that is contaminated by pathogenic microorganisms.

Culture:

a controlled population of growing microorganisms that is maintained for purposes of study. A pure culture contains only one type or strain of microorganism. Sampling of the hospital environment (surface or air) results in the obtaining of a "mixed" culture containing numerous microbial types. Individual colonies must be "isolated" from such mixed cultures for further study or identification.

Decontaminate:
to remove pathogenic and undesirable microorganisms or soil from surfaces by chemical or physical means.

Detergent:
a chemical used for cleaning surfaces, that may possess various properties such as surface wetting, soil emulsification, soil dispersion or soil suspending.

Disease:
the impairment of bodily health; illness or sickness; an "infectious disease" is caused by a pathogenic microorganism. A "contagious disease" is transmitted by contact with an infected person.

Disinfectant detergent:
a chemical product formulated with cleaning agents and germicides selected for soil removal and simultaneous disinfection. Disinfectant literally means "frees from infection," but generally is used as a synonym for germicide.

Disinfection:
the process of killing specific microorganisms by a physical or chemical means.

Droplet infection:
an infection produced by microorganisms carried in liquid droplets sometimes caused by a sneeze from an infected person. The aerosol produced by an aerator in a faucet contaminated with *pseudomonas* bacteria could contain droplets, which might spread this pathogenic bacteria and cause a droplet infection.

Dwell time:
contact time.

Emulsification:
lifting the soils of the surface and suspending them so they may be rinsed off.

Epidemic:

an unusually large number of cases of infection or disease within a given population. In contrast to "endemic," which refers to the "normal" state of a usual number of cases of infection or disease within a given population.

Epidemiology:

the study and investigation of the source, transmission, control, and prevention of contagious diseases and infections.

Fimbri:

anchoring strands of bacteria.

Flagellum:

a tail or whip used by bacteria to move around.

Fogging:

the practice of generating an aerosol of microscopic droplets less than ten microns in diameter. Such micro-droplets of disinfectant solutions are not capable of wetting surfaces and consequently do not produce sufficient antimicrobial activity either in the air or on environmental surfaces to depend on this practice for environmental decontamination.

Fomite:

any inanimate surface that is contaminated with infectious microorganisms that may transmit disease.

Fungi: (sing., fungus):

microscopic plants capable of growing either on dead organic matter as saprophytes or in living hosts as parasites (athlete's foot fungus). Although microscopic in size, fungi grow on surfaces to the extent that fluffy or powdery colonies can be seen without magnification.

Fungicide:

a chemical that kills or destroys fungal growth. Not all germicides may function as fungicides, nor do all fungicides act as germicides.

Gas gangrene:

an infection caused by a spore-forming bacillus—*clostridium perfringens* or *Cl. welchii*. The spores cannot be destroyed with most liquid germicides, but can be killed by heat sterilization.

Germ:

a common term for pathogenic bacteria or other microorganisms.

Germicide:

a chemical that destroys vegetative bacteria, but not necessarily the resistant spore form of bacteria. Not the same as "sterilize."

Gram:

a unit of weight measure in the metric system. There are 28.36 grams in an ounce.

Gram's stain:

a method of staining bacteria with various dyes for microscopic examination, invented by Christian Gram in 1884. Some bacteria when exposed to the stains will retain a blue dye (gram positive), whereas others will not (gram negative). The various bacterial types may be divided into two basic groups depending upon their reactions to the dyes used in this staining method.

Hanson's Disease:
another name for leprosy.

Hardness:

an expression of the concentration of inorganic salts in water that prevents effective cleaning and germicidal action. Hardness is measured in parts per million (ppm) calculated as calcium carbonate ($CaCo_3$).

Host:

any organism (man, animal, or plant) that acts as a growth site for parasitic microorganisms.

Hydrolysis:
when cleaning agents react with soils, particularly the facts that may be present, and then converting the soils to soap.

Immunity:
resistance to disease or infection because of body defenses or other physiological mechanisms. Immunology is the science of studying how resistance to disease or infection is developed or increased.

Inanimate:
without life.

Indirect transmission:
contracting a disease by touching a contaminated surface, then touching your eyes, mouth, or a mucous membrane.

Infection:
the entering of a microorganism and its subsequent growth within the host to produce the characteristics or symptoms of an infectious disease.

Iodophors:
modern version of iodine.

Isolate:
to restrict the movements of a patient with a communicable disease or infection so that cross-infection to other patients is prevented. Also, to protect a patient so that infectious microorganisms will not be brought into his/her area by other patients or staff members.

Leprosy:
a chronic infectious disease that attacks the skin, nerves, etc.; communicated after close, long contact.

Lysis:
the process of cell destruction whereby holes in the cell wall allow fluids to escape.

Microbes:
living organisms unseen by the naked eye; microorganisms.

Microbiology:
the branch of biology dealing with microorganisms.

Micron:
a unit of linear measure in the metric system. There are 25,400 microns in an inch. Bacteria usually measure about 1/2 micron in width and 5-10 microns in length.

Microorganisms:
living organisms unseen by the naked eye; microbes.

Multi-cellular:
made up of many cells.

Nonionic detergent:
a type of chemical that possesses surfactant properties including surface-wetting, and soil dispersion. This detergent chemical does not ionize with positive or negative charges. It is compatible in mixtures with either cationic or anionic surfactants. It is not compatible, however, with phenolic germicides.

Opportunistic microorganisms:
microbes that take advantage of the present opportunity, such as infecting people when they cannot fight off a microbe.

Pasteurization:
heating liquid to a prescribed temperature for a specified time period to destroy disease-producing bacteria.

Pathogen:
a microorganism capable of producing an infection.

pH:
the measurement symbol used to express the degree of acidity or alkalinity. A pH of 1 expresses in extremely acid condition, while a pH of 14 is highly alkaline. The pH scale

runs from less than 1.0 to 14 and neutrality is centered at pH 7.00.

Phenol:

carbolic acid. Phenol is the basic constituent of the synthetic phenolic germicides, most of which have antimicrobial properties superior to phenol itself. Phenol is the standard against which synthetic phenolic germicides are compared when the phenol coefficient is calculated.

Phenol coefficient:

the result of comparing a phenolic germicide with carbolic acid (phenol) where the dilution of germicide killing the test bacteria in 10 minutes is divided by the dilution of phenol also killing the test bacteria in 10 minutes. The quotient number is the phenol coefficient.

Protozoan:

single-cell animals that are found in water, foods, blood, and body fluids.

Quarternary ammonium compound (quats):

a germicidal callonic surfactant chemical group typified by n-alkyl dimethyl benzyl ammonium chloride. There are many types of quarternary ammonium germicides as compared to the relatively few phenolic germicides commonly used in disinfectant detergents. Quarternaries (quats) are completely soluble in water, are odorless, and react with many malodor compounds to deodorize them.

Residual activity:

the inhibition of bacterial growth processes due to the presence of antimicrobial chemical residues on surfaces. Residual activity depends on high relative humidity at the cell-surface to bring the chemical residue into contact with essential portions of the bacterial cell. Residual activity in absorbent materials (fabrics) is a useful function of this concept, but such activity on hard surfaces is not considered meaningful by most authorities in bacteriology.

Sanitary:

a clean and hygienically safe condition.

Sanitized:

clean and free from germs.

Sanitizer:

to chemically or physically reduce a microbial population to a level judged safe by public health requirements. Technically, to sanitize means to reduce a bacterial population by 99 percent to 99.999 percent or better. Sanitize is not the same as disinfect.

Saponification:

see hydrolysis.

Sepsis:

a state of infection or contamination by pathogenic microorganisms.

Spirochetes (SPEYE ruh keets):

spiral-shaped bacterium.

Stasis:

the state of inhibition of microbial growth, (e.g. bacteriostasis, fungistasis).

Sterile:

the absence of viable microbial life.

Sterilization:

the complete destruction of living matter.

Surfactant (ser FAC tent):

the wetting agent.

Terminal disinfection:

cleaning and decontamination procedures employed to destroy pathogenic bacteria within an area (isolation patient's room) to prevent cross-infection to others entering the area. Normally done with established procedures by personnel trained in the technique, after the discharge or removal of the patient from isolation.

Tetanus:
a disease caused by the infectious spore-forming bacteria *clostridium tetani*. Commonly referred to as lockjaw.

Tissue culture:
the growing of human or animal cells in a layer of single-cell thickness within a sterile container to furnish a living substrate for the culturing of certain viruses.

Tuberculocidal:
the ability to kill the tuberculosis bacteria under controlled laboratory conditions.

Tuberculosis:
an infectious disease that is characterized b y forming tubercles in tissues of the body.

Turbidity:
visible sign of microbial growth in liquid broth culture tubes or flasks.

Ultraviolet light (UV):
the range in the light spectrum between 3900 angstroms. The radiations in the range between 2000 and 2950 angstroms are germicidal to most bacteria.

Universal precautions:
the practice of treating everyone as if they are infected since it is impossible to tell if they are infected by merely looking at them.

Vegetative:
the actively growing stage of a bacterial cell as contrasted to the spore stage. Relatively few bacteria produce the spore stage.

Viable:
alive.

Virulence:
the degree of pathogenicity of an infectious microorganism.

Virus:

an infectious agent small enough in size to pass through filters that trap bacteria. Viruses cannot be seen with an ordinary light microscope, but can be observed with electron microscopes. Viruses must be cultured in living cells rather than in artificial culture medium.

References

Accreditation Manual for Hospitals, Joint Commission of Hospital Accreditation, Chicago, 1991.

Alyeffe, G. A. J. "Equipment-Related Infection Risks." *Journal of Hospital Infection.* Vol. 11, Supplement A, pgs. 279–284, 1988.

American Practitioners of Infection Control Curriculum Guide, 1990.

Ascenzi, J. M. "Standardization of Tuberculocidal Testing of Disinfectants." *Journal of Hospital Infection.* 18:256–263, 1991.

Babb, J. R. "Methods of Reprocessing Complex Medical Equipment." *Journal of Hospital Infection.* Supplement A, pgs. 285–291, 1988.

Bennett, J. V., and P. S. Brachman. *Hospital Infections.* 3rd ed. Boston: Little, Brown. 1992.

Block, S. S. *Disinfection, Sterilization, and Preservation.* 4th ed. Philadelphia: Lea and Ferberger. 1992.

Branson D. "The Other Mycobacteria." *Remel Microbiology Newsletter.* Vol. 3, No. 1, pgs. 65–70, 1985.

Burnbaum, J. "Urban Plagues." *Mirabella.* pgs. 132–134, March 1992.

Burnstein, P. "Hepatitis B." *Cosmopolitan.* pgs. 124–126, June 1992

Chesky, S. "In Line Validation of Sanitizing Agents in the Aseptic Core." *Journal of Perenteral Science.* 1986

Ching, T. Y. and W. H. Seto. "Hospital Use of Chlorine Disinfectants in a Hepatitis B Endemic Area ...." *Journal of Hospital Infection.* 14:39–47, 1989.

Christiansen, R., R. A. Robinson, D. F. Robinson, B. J. Ploeger, R. W. Leavitt and H. L. Bodily. "Antimicrobial Activity of Environmental Surface Disinfectants in the Absence and Presence of Bioburden." *Journal of the American Dental Association.* 119:493–505, October 1989.

Cristina, Isabel. *Proper Disinfection for the Beauty Industry: Protecting Yourself While Protecting Your Clients.* VHS format video. 40 minutes. Teaneck, NJ: RBR Productions, Inc., 1992.

Cundy, K. R. et al. *Infection Control Dilemmas and Practical Solutions.* New York: Plenum Press, 1990.

Danforth, D., et. al. "Nosocomial Infections on Nursing Units with Floors Cleaned with a Disinfectant Compared with Detergent." *Journal of Hospital Infection.* 10:229–235, 1987.

Dewar, N. E. *Phenolic Disinfecting.*

Disinfectants, Soaps/Cosmetics/Chemical Specialties. pgs. 26–27, 84–86, December 1988.

Dodd, R. and F. Lewellys. (eds.) *Infections, Immunity, and Blood Transfusion.* 1985.

du Moulin, G. C. and K. D. Stottmeier. *Waterborne Mycobacteria: An Increasing Threat to Health.* ASM News. Vol. 52, No. 10, pgs. 525–529, 1986.

Engley, F. "Asepsis, Disinfection, and Sterilization in Health Care Facilities." *Infection Control: A Policy and Procedure Manual*, Chem Bio, Milwaukee, Wisconsin. 1978.

Favaro, M., *Letters on Hazards of the Gram-Negative Water Bacteria,* Center for Disease Control, Atlanta, GA.

Fine, P. E. M. and L. C. Rodriges. *Microbacterial Diseases,* Lancet Publishing, 335:1016–1020, April 28, 1990.

Fox, J. D., M. Briggs, P. A. Ward and Tedder. "Human Herpes Virus 6 in Salivary Glands." *The Lancet.* Vol. 336, No. , pgs. 590–593, September 1990.

Geden, C. J. "Efficacies of Mixtures of Disinfectants and Insecticides." *Poultry Science.* 66:659–665, 1987.

"Germicides, Disinfectants, and Antimicrobials: Will Government Force Us Back to Bucket and Scrub Brush?" *Chemical Purchasing,* May 1979.

Good Hospital Practice: Handling and Biological Decontamination of Reusable Medical Devices, American National Standard, Association for the Advancement of Medical Instrumentation. ANSI/AAMI, March 1991.

Groschel, D. H. M. "Disinfectant Testing in the USA." *Journal of Hospital Infection.* Vol. 18, Supplement A, pgs 274–279, 1991.

Guidelines for Prevention of Transmission of Human Immunodeficiency Virus and Hepatitis B Virus to Health-Care Report, Atlanta, Vol. 38, No. 5–6, June 23, 1989.

Horowitz, E. A. "Recent Trends in Mycobacterial Diseases." *Hospital Formulary.* 23:892–897, November 1988.

Hotchkin, J. *Slow Virus Diseases.* 1974.

"Infection Control Recommendations for the Dental Office and the Dental Laboratory." *Journal of the American Dental Association.* Vol. 116, February 1988.

Jacoby, G. A. and G. L. Archer. "New Mechanisms of Bacterial Resistance to Antimicrobial Agents." *The New England Journal of Medicine.* Vol. 324, No. 9, pgs. 601–612, February 28, 1991.

Jawetz E., J. L. Melnick and E. A. Adelberg. *Review of Medical Microbiology.* 15th ed. New York: Lange Medical Publications. 1982.

Jonsson, V. M. "An Easy Step-by-Step Method of Selecting Hospital Disinfectants." *Executive Housekeeping Today.* September 12, 1988.

Karim, Q. N. et. al. "Routine Cleaning and the Elimination of Campylobacter Pylori from Endoscopic Biopsy Forceps." *Journal of Hospital Infection.* 13:87–90, 1989.

Kerr, K. G. and R. W. Lacey. "Listeriosisi: New Problems with an Old Pathogen," *Journal of Hospital Infection.* 12:247–250, 1988.

Kolari, P. J., et. al. "Cleansing of Hands with Emulsion—A Solution to Skin Problems of Hospital Staff." *Journal of Hospital Infection.* 13:377–386, 1989.

Kunin, C., D. Bauer and F. Engley. "Choosing a Nursery Disinfectant." *Hospital Infection Control*, April 1980.

Litsky, B. Y. *Hospital Sanitation.* Chicago: Clissold Publishing Company, 1966.

Lund, B. M. "Foodborne Disease Due to Bacillus and Clostridium Species." *The Lancet.* 336:982–986, 1990.

Lund, B. M. "Foodborne Illness." *The Lancet*, October 20, 1990.

Maki, D. G., C. J. Alvarado, C. A. Hassemer and M. A. Zilz. "Relation of the Inanimate Hospital Environment to Endemic Nosocomial Infection." *New England Journal of Medicine.* 307:1562, 1982.

Mallison, G. F. and R. W. Haley. "Microbial Sampling of the Inanimate Environment in U.S. Hospitals." *American Journal of Medicine.* 70:941, 1981.

Martyr, Hamilton, Dr. and George A. Z. Karian. *Secretary-General's Comprehensive Report on Global Infection Control.*

Geneva, Switzerland: UN World Health Organization, 1993.

Mbithi, J. N., V. S. Springthorpe and S. A. Sattar. *Chemical Disinfection of Hepatitis A Virus on Environmental Surfaces, Applied and Environmental Microbiology.* Vol. 56, No. 11, pgs. 3601–3604, November 1990.

Meyer, R. D. and R. G. Finch. "Community-Acquired Pneumonia." *Journal of Hospital Infection.* Vol. 22, 1992.

Monmaney, T. and P. McKillop. "The Return of Tuberculosis." *Newsweek*, pg. 68, February 22, 1988.

Naides, S. J., "Infection Control Measures for Human Parvovirus B19 in the Hospital Setting." *Infection Control Hospital Epidemiology.* Vol. 10, No. 7, pgs. 326–329, 1988.

1990 Medical and Health Annual. Encyclopedia Britannica Inc. Chicago, Illinois.

Physical Properties of Particles. SRI International, Menlo Park, CA, USA.

Policy Statements, American Public Health Association, October 25, 1989, *American Journal of Public Health*, Vol. 80, No. 2, February 1990.

Prince, H. N. *Disinfectant Activity Against Bacteria and Viruses: A Hospital Guide, Particulate and Microbial Control.* March/April 1983.

Proposed Recommended Practices, Steam and Ethylene Oxide Sterilization. American Society for Central Service, Vol. 55, No. 1, January 1992.

A Review of Disinfectants, Part II. Infection Control Rounds, Vol. 4, No. 1, March 1980.

Reybrouck, G. "International Standardization of Disinfectant Testing—Is It Possible?" *Journal of Hospital Infection.* Vol. 18, Supplement A, pgs. 280–288, 1991.

Rosenberg, Richard Benjamin. *Product Data Report on Current Disinfection Methods*. Teaneck, NJ: RBR Productions. 1990.

Rosenberg, Richard Benjamin. "State Boards and the Future of the Beauty Industry: For National Disinfection for the 90s." *NIC (National-Interstate Council of Boards of Cosmetology) Bulletin*. 3:October 1992.

Russell, A. D., W. B. Hugo and G. A. J. Alyffe. (eds.) *Principles and Practice of Disinfection, Preservation, and Sterilization*. Great Britain: Blackwell Scientific Publications. 1982.

Rutala, W. A. "APIC Guideline for the Selection and Use of Disinfectants." *American Journal of Infection Control*, Vol. 17, No. 52, pgs. 99–117, 1990.

Simmons, B., et. al. "Infection Control for Home Health." *Infection Control Hospital Epidemiology*. 11:362–370, 1990.

Spaulding, E. H. and E. K. Emmons. "Chemical Disnfection." Paper presented at Seton Hall College of Medicine and Dentistry as part of the Becton Dickenson Series, April 1, 1958.

Spaulding, E. H., *Principles and Application of Chemical Disinfection. Aorn Journal*, Vol. 1, No. 3, May–June 1963.

Tyler, R., G. A. J. Alyiffe and C. Bradley. "Virucidal Activity of Disinfectants: Studies with the Poliovirus." *Journal of Hospital Infection*. 15:339–345, 1990.

U.S. Government, EPA Definitions, DIS/TSS–1, January, 1979.

Warren, R. E. "Difficult Streptococci." *Journal of Hospital Infection*. Vol. 22, Supplement A, pgs 352–357, 1988.

Yearbook of Medicine. Mosby, Missouri: 1990, 1991, and 1992.